Is There A Doctor In The Country?

*****

Copyright © 2014 by Tanya L. Taylor

Revised 2016

"Silent Illness," is an unfamiliar condition with multiple names like Gastroparesis, Digestive Tract Paralysis, Ehlers-Danlos, Dysautonomia, Mast Cell Activation Disorders, and Chiari Malformation.

These names are unknown to most, but many are diagnosed with one or more illnesses out of this group of Silent Illnesses. In the medical community, a person may have to see many specialists, and go through frightening procedures before they get a diagnosis, a name. Worse yet, these illnesses have no known cures, and are more common than you would think. The confusion, pain, and suffering Tanya L. Taylor has lived through, was not easy to talk about for a long time. Now, she wants to make sure her voice, and the voices of those trying to live with these devastating illnesses, are heard.

Tanya has decided to BREAK THE SILENCE. In this book, she shares her medical journey of mis-diagnoses, frustration and *faith*.

Table of Contents

Foreword

I was 43 years old when I first began writing this book. A lifetime of painful illness, going from bad to worse, created lots of questions. There were many answers I was given; most of which were totally incorrect, flawed or inaccurate. Some even fictitious with little correct information and many more questions. I didn't know what else to do other than write, describe my symptoms, and ask "Is There a Doctor in the Country?"

I wanted to know why all of these horrible things I was living with were happening prior to being diagnosed with Gastroparesis (GP). No one could tell me anything. I was passed from one doctor to another through the Johns Hopkins GI medical groups. I was in and out of a GI Group in Towson, MD at GBMC (Greater Baltimore Medical Center). My personal physician, who I will refer to as Dr. X, from Overlea Personal Physicians, also had me seeing specialists at

Mercy Hospital in Baltimore, MD. I was not getting any answers from anyone as to why I was so sick, throwing up, and losing so much weight. It is imperative to remember that each physician is human, with his or her own personality. It is important not to give credit to a physician, simply because of the name of a hospital or University. Not every physician is educated or knowledgeable about many illnesses in the world of Silent Illnesses.

I was almost finished writing my book when I learned that I had Gastroparesis, a Silent Illness with chronic and potentially life threatening digestive issues with no known cure. By this time, I had lost my colon and gall bladder. If I had learned that I had GP years earlier, would I still have those organs? Would I be healed or feeling better? Perhaps. However, that is not the purpose of this book.

My intention for writing this is to assure others with these type of Silent Illnesses they are not alone. In addition, my *hope* is that each person is able to find something that will provide them with *hope*, be able to live stronger, and help one another. I know they say there is no cure, but I do not believe it has to stay that way. I am trying to find a way to help myself while those working in the medical field try to understand and find a cure for these illnesses.

I had to fight hard for my life early in 2008. I almost died from septicemia, due to bacteria that had perforated through my colon into my bloodstream. That happened just prior to the removal of my colon on March 20, 2008. I was in ICU for a few days. I was able to go to a regular room after finding the proper antibiotics in which I was responding well to and was able to walk to the bathroom by myself. When I walked in and saw my reflection in the mirror, I let out a scream in horror. My skin was gray. I looked like a zombie from those movies. That was the first, among many life battles I have had to fight. This particular sepsis is the only time I turned gray. Septicemia from the IV nutrition lines is a battle in itself, but the battle from our waste system - the intestines - is a battle I do not want to face again, and much more difficult to fight.

In addition to my colon ceasing to function, I had to live with a life line for nutrition that was supplied through my veins called TPN (Total Parenteral Nutrition) also known as IV nutrition. I was unable to eat anymore because the food would no longer move through my system. For me, this did not happen overnight. It took years, decades to be exact. For others, they are born with this in an extreme form and have to live off of TPN or J Tube feedings. J Tube feedings come from a tube that is placed through the wall of the stomach, into the jejunum part of the small intestine. Nutrients are absorbed in the small intestine, while fluids are absorbed in the large intestine. It is important that the body receives nutrients and fluids through the IV

Many physicians told me this was in my head because they could not figure it out. No one seemed to know what was going on, and I was tired of being called names like "whiny woman," "baby," and/or "drug seeker." I was so tired of being made fun of and being told that this was in my head. One doctor said to me during one visit, "You are dying right in front of me, but I don't know what to do." This same doctor who, a couple of years later, kicked me out of GBMC and told me my tests were cancelled. She told me that I would do better with a different group of physicians. Prior to this action, I was being accused of being a Demerol seeker, as usual, because of my allergies to everything else.

I was sent to Philadelphia, PA, to Temple University in the later months of 2007. Many medical diagnoses were found during the 2007-2008 visits, but I was not informed about any of this information, including the diagnosis of Gastroparesis. When I landed in Georgetown

University Hospital in DC mid-2011, the records from Temple University were ordered and I was informed at that time that I had Gastroparesis. Further down the road in October of 2012, I ended up finding other medical diagnoses while reviewing my own medical records. I was not informed of any of this, in addition to the GP diagnosis in 2008. During one of my visits in 2005, Dr. X had documentation then that I had Gastroparesis neglecting to mention this to me or provide me with any information about the diagnosis. I had to figure out on my own why I felt so horrible.

I was never taken seriously growing up about how horrible I felt. At home, I was always made to push through pain and whatever symptoms I was having. I never looked as bad as I felt which should not have been a factor. I was complaining all of the time about my stomach. I've had knots in my neck and back since elementary school. I had to have the knots massaged daily if I was going to be able to turn my head or be able to move around. I learned to continue my day no matter how I felt. No one in my family listened when I told them how sick I was. No one listened when I told them my stomach hurt, or that it had been days since I had gone to the bathroom. Everyone thought I was making it up, or that I wasn't feeling as bad as I said I was. Why didn't they believe me? Was it because I could still run around trying to still be a kid? I will never really know. Even in the eyes of my family there was nothing wrong with me.

Regardless of how sick I was or wasn't, someone should have listened to me when I told them I wasn't feeling well. If someone tells you they are not feeling well, and you cannot see what they are feeling; then do not assume they are not telling the truth because you are unable to see or feel what that person is going through. Lives have been lost prematurely because of critical harsh judgments and lack of care.

I had to change this entire book after researching and finding new knowledge about this illness. I went from looking for a doctor, to educating about Gastroparesis. I will touch on other illnesses that have been diagnosed in addition to Gastroparesis. More in depth information will be given in, "Is There a Doctor in the Country? Volume 2." There are several medical issues that are not related but seem to run together. While someone with Gastroparesis may only have complications due to GP, others may be suffering with other illnesses that make life even more difficult. GP is a devastating, debilitating illness that needs much more attention than the medical profession and government has allowed. It is through the federal government that laws for research need to be passed. The government has to recognize that this is a serious issue affecting the lives of millions by taking the time to hear bills, and passing legislation. Otherwise those living and dying with these Silent Illnesses will continue to fight in the dark. Since the government has so much control over this issue, the government and the National Institute of Health (NIH) should be making this a priority. The lives of millions in the U.S., as well as so many abroad, depend on people becoming educated.

It is time the medical professionals be held accountable for the care of others. Doctors are people who went to school trying to figure out life, just like the rest of us who are not physicians. Doctors are not above the law, above you or me, and certainly not above God. God gifts miracles, we are merely vessels. Through life's journey, we figure out, or realize that there is no one person more important or better than anyone else. While we are not all treated equal, we are all equal and deserve the same "Right to Life." Those who are born with debilitating diseases or illnesses deserve to live a full life just like those without such challenges. One disease or illness is not worse than another when it comes to chronic illness.

Devastation due to illness is devastation. A person with any chronic illness should not have to go through the judgment other people have as to which illness is worse. Each medical condition is not only devastating to the person who is inflicted by it, but to those who are friends and family of the person who is sick. One disease or illness should not receive preferential treatment because of stardom or popularity. All chronic illness is horrible. How can anyone sit in judgment if they have not experienced what they are judging? **Judgments need to stop so that education and healing can begin.**

Editor's Note

The first time I met Tanya L. Taylor, in person, I was shocked by what I saw. A day or two after she missed an appointment with me, I reached her on her cell. She was ill and in a nearby hospital. I decided to go see her. After all, she didn't sound sick; maybe I could do something to help.

Walking into that hospital room was the first step of a new friendship. Although at the moment I first saw her, I didn't think she had long to live. She was thin, pale, grasping herself in pain, gasping for breath, and hooked up to tubes and monitors. When she described a tiny bit of her undiagnosed condition and listed organs she had lost, I started to drift off in thought. I wondered if there was anything I could do. I decided I would be company, distraction, and a good listener.

Over the course of that hospital stay, I visited a few times. I saw her argue for a drug at the dose she knew, from experience, would work for her pain. I saw Tanya be denied that relief. "They see me as a drug seeker. I am not a seeker." Who was right? I didn't know her that well.

This hospital had certain rules about the drug dosage. She couldn't change their minds. As much as I was sympathetic to her suffering, those in the white coats had field advantage. Even if it was "all in her head," she was in dire-straights physically. Didn't she deserve more help?

Nurses did what they could. I listened as hospital doctors and interns would visit with Tanya. It seemed like the usual looking at charts and asking her some questions. One of her own doctors stopped in, apparently didn't like the conversation and dismissed herself from the case. Tanya's comments to me after these visits: "No one knows what this is" and "I've been told it is all in my head."

It was beautiful that week in May of 2011. I came into Tanya's hospital room with some energized water for her. It was near the end of her stay. She was remarkably brighter. She was busy on her lap top. She was making calls. She had "rallied to the cause." It was a day before the weekend event, The World of Possibilities Expo. The table space for her non-profit would be without her. On top of that, the scheme to raise money was fouled by a photographer who backed out of his job that day. She was desperately trying to find a replacement. She knew the money raised would help young families. Her focus had turned outward again.

Her cause now includes you, the reader. Is There a Doctor In The Country? is a result of her rallying again. Certainly she wants to improve her health. Each day is a challenge to get out of bed. Push back the pain. Deal with friends and family affected by her illness. All of which is physically and emotionally draining for anyone with any illness.

In these pages, you get the benefit of Tanya's persistent research on Silent Illnesses. Her seemingly endless quest for medical professionals, knowledgeable and willing enough to take on her case. Her voice has brought awareness to Gastroparesis, Ehlers-Danlos and more. Her open discussion of family challenges may help explain the conflicts and provide some advice for coping. You'll know why you must always question the details when it comes to your health.

As I see it, a part of what keeps Tanya alive is desire to serve others. The other big part is her craving to get back her life. Much of what she has learned has come with a loss of pieces, not only the body parts, but pieces of relationships, dreams, independence, time, opportunity and occasionally, even her strong *faith* and *hope*.

What you may find in these pages could be knowledge, *hope*, belief, courage, anger, appreciation, gratitude or something else you've needed.

What is my takeaway from Is There a Doctor in the Country? I could have been one who judged her. Early in our friendship, she would tell me about the labels she'd been given -- drug seeker, or doctor jumper, mentally unstable. I trusted my gut and am very glad I did. I can see now how medical biases, professional ego, or a note on the referring doctor's report, may have contributed to how she was viewed and treated.

Tanya L Taylor, is a loving, caring person with a broad range of important information and experience to relate. I am so glad I took the time to know her as my friend.

Tanya's advice for us all: Don't stand in judgment.

Pam Gecan

Chapter 1

Septic

I'll never forget the morning I went septic. My husband, Mike, had already left for work. I started getting some strength back because of the iv nutrition line the doctor placed. I decided I would throw some laundry in. While I was downstairs, I started feeling so strange. I was getting dizzy, weak, and then I couldn't think straight. I was freezing cold and began shaking so badly I could barely push the start button before going back upstairs to my bed. I could feel my body drowning in fever, and with every second, I was feeling worse.

When I got myself up to my bed, I yelled for my daughter. My daughter, Samantha, was home the morning I became septic. Thank God! She was about 7 months pregnant and she came running into my room. When she saw me, she was afraid and didn't know what to do. I asked her to call Mike. Let him know what was happening to me, and tell him to turn around and come right back home. I had her turn on the heating pad, cover me with blankets, put the heating pad on top of the blankets and lay on top of me. The convulsion type shaking from the spike in fever had my body in so much pain I could barely tolerate it.

I didn't know at that point I was septic and needed medical attention ASAP. Sam stayed on top of me while we waited for Mike to come home. She tried to help me get the uncontrollable movements to calm. The pain from those types of fever shakes takes every muscle in my back, neck, and hips so out of control I can hardly stand it. We ended up driving to GBMC, a hospital approximately 40 minutes away from our home. I was born at GBMC. I didn't know where else to go. My doctors were in Baltimore County, about 30 miles north of where I moved when I married Mike.

I was admitted into the hospital, into the glass room where everyone watches your every breath. ICU. I did not want to be there. I remember when my husband's family came into the hospital and looked at me, their faces were that of shock. I couldn't understand why they were looking at me the way they were. I just knew I wanted the doctors to find out what was going on and get me out of that hospital. After the cultures were developed, and they knew which antibiotic to administer, I began to get better.

It took a couple of days of being in the hospital, in that glass room, before I was able to be moved to a regular room. It was so wonderful when that day came. I couldn't wait to get away from the glass room. When I was taken to my new room, where I didn't have to be monitored every second, I got out of the bed they wheeled me from, and went into the bathroom. It felt so good to walk on my own.

As I walked into the bathroom, I saw myself in the mirror for the first time in a few days. I was so frightened by what I saw I screamed. I was gray. My skin was actually the color gray. I looked like a zombie from one of those zombie movies. I looked like a walking corpse. Mike came running into the bathroom while I was standing in disbelief and horror at what I was seeing. I started to cry showing and telling him I was gray and looked like I was dead. He said, "No, you look good." I looked good? What did I look like before? I cannot even imagine. No wonder everyone who knew me, and saw me, looked at me with that face. The face of, "Oh my God!"

Prior to becoming septic, I had been in and out of the hospital, emergency room, and doctors' offices for decades. No one seemed to know what was going on other than female issues, so automatically I was labeled depressed and anxious. They were not seeing that the colon was dying and that I was in terrible pain from the food not moving through properly. I wasn't feeling well from not receiving the proper nutrition and hydration the way people with a "normal" digestive system are able to do. Even though I continued to push on as I was taught to as a child, I was always feeling worn out quicker than others.

When you are sick your entire life, not feeling well and your family doesn't seem to hear what you are saying, you have two choices; learn to adapt, or miss out on life. I chose to adapt to the pain and illness from this body I was trapped in. Digestive issues plagued me all the way back to preschool years, as well as having horrible colic when I was a baby. I started developing a fear of hospitals and doctors in my early thirties. I was given so many drugs that made me sick or could have killed me, in addition to the horrible attitudes of judgment and lack of medical care. I feel very blessed to still be alive. I know that God has been making sure that all of this has not killed me, so that I am able to write this book and speak out for those who live the way I have and are unable to speak out.

After I was discharged from the hospital, it was time to find a surgeon to remove my colon. Temple University had already found Colonic Inertia, which means my colon was not functioning properly. During the hospital stay, it was apparent that the colon was more of a threat to my life, than a help. The discussion about the colon was the same with the doctors in the hospital. Dr. X told me that I should keep my colon and not have it removed. He also stated that the IV nutrition I was on was unnecessary because I did not want to eat - not that my body was not allowing me to eat. My colon at this time was killing me, and instead of Dr. X listening to what I was telling him, he told me to keep the colon. What? I don't think so! I had the surgery done regardless of his opinion.

I cannot stress enough the importance of advocating for yourself with any type of issue, medical or not. You know what your body is feeling. I could feel my colon dying the entire time. For years I had been saying that it needed to be removed and no one listened to me. I knew there was something seriously wrong. The years of pain I suffered, while it was dying, is just unconscionable to know there was no one educated enough to know what was happening to me. I did not receive proper medical care the entire time I was explaining what was happening, and I didn't receive proper medical care after the January 9, 2008 medical reports diagnosing Gastroparesis. Did Dr. X decide he was not going to be bothered with reading my medical records sent to him from Temple University? Those medical records had vital information that showed I am a Poor Metabolizer. I have Gastroparesis in addition to the Colonic Inertia. Colonic Inertia seems to be a very common problem for those who have Gastroparesis.

###

Psalms 46:1-2

God is our refuge and strength [mighty and impenetrable], A very present and well-proved help in trouble. Therefore will we not fear, though the earth should change, And though the mountains be shaken and slip into the heart of the seas,

Chapter 2

Medical Excuses and Labels

Digestive Tract Paralysis has been known about for decades, yet medical professionals were not educated enough to help me through this. Instead, I was labeled a Drug Seeker. I was the drug seeker because the doctors could not figure out what was going on and refused to believe I was suffering in pain, along with the inability to eat. Having a genetic condition known as "Poor Metabolism," my body is unable to tolerate so many types of medication, including narcotics, with the exception of Demerol. Demerol is an old school narcotic that I have absolutely no side effects from. I don't feel drugged and I don't feel sleepy. My pain just reduces to a degree that I can tolerate it.

I was told by doctors my pain was from addiction or was in my head. Oh yes, and of course, one of the other common questions that always came up was, "Is she making herself vomit?" At two separate times, when I ended up having to have Botox injections of the pyloric area, the vomiting turned into projectile vomiting. I guess I must have learned the puke talent quite well to turn it into projective vomiting.

Living this life has been nothing short of frustrating with the medical profession. I always told doctors exactly what I was feeling, but it was as if no one could hear the words I was saying. Instead, according to the medical notes I've been reading from doctors' visits, the two big questions are, "Is this psychosomatic?" and "Is she forcing herself to throw up?" So, instead of taking my time and my money to help me, many physicians decided to judge my health based on their own discriminatory thoughts and opinions of previous patients, or their own personal experiences, and bill me for their uneducated judgmental harsh behaviors and comments.

It is not a win/win situation out here with the medical profession/patient relationship in the United States. Since many doctors do not listen to their patients, and medications are prescribed that a person should not take for various reasons, there should be a system that is keeping track of the information about the effects of each drug on each patient.

During the First Health Care Summit, held at the U.S. Chamber of Commerce in October 2012, I was in attendance and took notes as quickly as I could so I would get as much info as possible. I do a great deal of research, and was so fortunate to be out of the hospital, on my feet, and at that Summit. During the first half of that day, a great deal of my research was confirmed, in addition to learning other information I had not found yet. One of the facts brought up during the Summit was that the U.S. has only a 55% success ratio of patient/physician relationships. Meaning, out of 100% of those in the study, only 55% of the patients who actually receive healthcare, have the care that is meant for them to be able to live happy healthy lives. Almost half of those who receive care in the U.S. do not receive the type of care that allows them to live life to the fullest, despite ailments.

Part of the data used in this statistic includes a patient's "willingness" to take drugs prescribed, as it is prescribed by the doctor. Whether or not a person has an adverse reaction to the medication is not in question. The responsibility of the faulty health care system is being laid at the feet of patients, more so than the feet of the physicians. When I think of the data being used to determine a successful relationship, I cannot help but be more alarmed and even more certain that the 55% success ratio that was discussed during the Summit is too high. Even with the 55% figure suggested, 45% of those in the United States will live with health issues that may be life threatening, as I am, and not receive the health care needed to stay alive or even live a functional life. The data regarding a patient's compliance pertaining to the use of drugs prescribed, cannot be accurate in any way and should be excluded from that study, or modified to indicate adverse reactions. By tracking drugs, and not tracking the sensitivities and allergies, any data collected would create false statistical results. False in this case meaning the statistic being used is skewed too high due to inaccurate information.

Gastroparesis can be excruciatingly painful, however, too many physicians have told me and many other GPers I know that GP does not cause pain. That is one of the craziest things I have heard a doctor say about this illness. I would like to know where they are reading this information they are using and who is teaching this. Do any of the doctors who say it does not cause pain have Gastroparesis and know what it actually feels like? The pain, when food sits in your system for days, while the cells are ceasing to function, is equivalent to what you would see in a war movie where soldiers are being cut without sedative or numbing agents. Where no matter what you do, there is no escaping the pain and exhaustion. Imagine being operated on while awake, without being numb, and expected to lay there without making a sound. The expectation is that those of us living with Gastroparesis should just "deal" with this degree of suffering I see on a daily basis. This life is like a roller coaster ride, so the pain can be over a ten one minute, using a scale of one to ten, and down to five the next. Every moment I see judgment with how someone thinks we feel.

The medical community, where there is not enough education about this debilitating illness and related illnesses, is where I, and millions of people with GP, Ehlers-Danlos (EDS), Dysautonomia, and other medical issues common to Gastroparesis, are trying to seek help and count on physicians who know very little about these types of Silent Illnesses, and don't seem to want to know. I am not discrediting those who are working to understand what is happening and what they can do to help. I am making a point that there are a multitude of physicians who do not understand the illnesses compared to one physician who does. We want more physicians to learn what is happening, be held accountable for learning about this group of Silent Illnesses so that those of us suffering are not pushed aside and treated like we have three heads. We are all surviving life the best we know how and deserve the compassion, understanding, and knowledge of the medical community. Many of us with Gastroparesis, Ehlers-Danlos Syndrome, and other Silent Illnesses, do not receive compassion and understanding. We do not receive that support that is so needed. As a matter of fact, many of us get the exact opposite which creates unnecessary stress and an unnecessary increase in pain, nausea, and further complications.

While the medical community sees us as just a patient, I see a patient as the one employing those working in the medical profession. I don't see the medical profession paying our bills; I see us paying the bills of those in the medical profession and our expenses increasing. If I am paying for a service, regardless of what that service is, retail or medical, I expect to get what I am paying for. If I am paying a physician in a special field, I expect that the physician be educated in his or her field. I've grown weary of the excuses doctors and medical staff give to hide behind. I've grown weary of hearing "I don't know." Well, no one else is permitted to hide behind "I don't know." If you have a tax due or court date, you better not give the excuse, "I didn't know." A judge will give you NO room for excuse, nor will the IRS. So why is it when it comes to our life, which I find to be much more important than a missed court date or a tax bill, the medical profession is allowed to say, "I don't know." I wish someone would explain that logic to me, because my brain cannot absorb it. If I am paying for a service, and I have paid for decades to be told it was all in my head until I almost died, who is going to reimburse me and make this entire situation right?

I've spoken to a number of attorneys to find we don't have the rights we should. Since there is not a permanent devastation that can be seen with their eyes, we have no rights and the funds aren't enough for an attorney to take on a fight without visual permanent damage. What about the visual permanent damage I have seen happen in my life day in and day out? What about the permanent damage it has caused my daughter to watch her mother be this sick and not be able to do anything about it? Why is it that I can be kicked out of an emergency room when I needed my gall bladder out immediately, while being accused of being a drug seeker, and forced to deal with an additional week of horrible intense pain, only to be admitted a week later to have a four hour surgery, which left me internally bleeding? Why do we as patients not have the right to protect ourselves from the judgments made by those in the medical field every day of the week?

It is very important for people who do not live with Silent Illnesses to begin to try to understand how much we suffer, and how their actions can impact how we feel. It is also very important for the front staff of a medical office to be compassionate, nice, smile, and be understanding. The opinions staff may hold about a person who is a patient is irrelevant. People in the forefront of medical offices have become so judgmental, that those who are seeking medical support have to come up against a lot of negative, nasty attitudes before ever seeing the physician. If someone chooses a profession in the medical field, as with a sales position or other people-oriented position, be prepared to smile and have a good day every day. Do not let those who have come in for help see the type of day you are having. It is important to put that smile on and welcome each patient who is also a client, with respect and dignity. Not attitude and disrespect. Somewhere those in the medical profession fail to see that their salaries, life styles, and business in general, are functioning because of the monies we, the patients, the clients, pay out for the health care we are asking to receive. We deserve the same courtesy and consideration as business owners give their customers, their clientele.

With that being said, in 2008, it was time to find a surgeon to remove my colon. My first surgery was at the age of 15, for a female illness called Endometriosis. I had to have surgeries each year to every other year from the Endometriosis. I had been through so much with my health with asthma, Endometriosis, and digestive issues by the time 2008 rolled around, I was frustrated and terrified of hospitals and doctors. No one believed me when I told them about my stomach problems with eating, and was forced to suffer in silence because of being turned away by numerous doctors and misdiagnosed with Depression.

Although I was afraid to have this surgery, I knew I had to have my colon removed if I was going to live. I had to make sure that whoever did this surgery was going to save my life. Someone who would make sure while he or she was removing my colon, that I did not become septic again, that I survived the surgery, that other organs were not harmed, and that I did not end up with a colostomy bag. I knew I was going to need the best. I found the best. You see, God is so great. I found Dr. Habibi.

Dr. Habibi cared. He knew this procedure was necessary. He felt compassion about the fact that I was young and he did not want to see me walking around with a colostomy bag. He knew that for me to have the best life I could, he had to do everything he could to make sure I did not end up with a bag. He did just that. He removed the colon. The entire thing was removed with the exception of a small bit where he attached the small intestine. He did it. He gave me a chance to figure out how to have a life with what I had left, and bought me time to live. He helped to give me time to find out what was wrong with me in the first place, time with my family, time to live.

###

Mark 11:25

And when you stand praying, if you hold anything against anyone, forgive him, so that your Father in heaven may forgive you your sins.

Chapter 3

Life Without a Colon

My colon was removed on March 20, 2008. I remember being anxious, but not overly fearful. I knew if the colon was not removed, that I could possibly become septic again. Septicemia was not a battle I wanted to fight a second time. My surgeon, Dr. Habibi, was a thoughtful communicator and spoke to me like a human being. He cared which helped give me a great deal of trust in having this surgery. We had multiple appointments to discuss all that would happen. Dr. Habibi wanted to make sure that I did not end up with a colostomy at the end of the surgery. I was only 41 when my colon was removed, so he looked at my life with consideration, and what I would have to deal with after the surgery was performed. He looked at me as a person, as well as a patient and not a number.

So many times in all areas of medicine that I have had to deal with, the majority of doctors were not very kind or considerate of what I was going through. More times than not, doctors would sit in judgment or disbelief, as if everything I was telling them was a lie.

I am allergic or oversensitive to almost all medications I have ever been given since I was born. Whether it is a controlled substance, anti-inflammatory, nausea medicine, or any other type of medicine you can think of, I generally cannot take them without having some kind of reaction.

Prior to the total Colectomy, my husband, Mike and I specifically told the doctors, and hospital staff, that I could not tolerate any type of pain medication with the exception of Demerol. After the surgery was over, I was placed on a Morphine drip. I barely remember anything for the two days they had me on this. Morphine has a negative effect on my respiratory system, creates hives, so it is not a medication that I should be given. I was given morphine a couple of times throughout the past 6 years. The last time they gave it to me, I ended up with respiratory issues once again.

During this surgery, I don't know if I had hives or not because I was unconscious. I had tubes coming from both nostrils to drain the blood and fluid from my stomach. I could do nothing. I remember coming-to once in a while, and the unbearable pain of the surgery. It was excruciating. It hurt to just be alive when I started to wake slightly. I remember Mike saying, "Push the button. Just push the button." I remember feeling him pushing my thumb on a button to give me the meds when I needed them. He was not allowed to push the button, but made sure to be there when I needed it. My brain couldn't think from the medicine and I couldn't open my eyes from the excruciating pain as well as the medicine. I was on the wrong meds which put me in a state of unconsciousness, at risk for additional complications, instead of pain relief.

I was still in a fog when the Occupational Therapist (OT) had come up to the room to talk to me and set up therapy sessions. The OT informed the nurses that there was no way she could work with me. She told them I was over-medicated and unable to respond. That gave my husband the opportunity to say, yet again, give her the Demerol and she will be fine. They finally switched my pain medication to the Demerol and I began to wake up. At that point, they had taken out the tubes. Mike and my mom were sitting on chairs to the right side of the foot of the hospital bed. I started to be able to focus and hear what was going on around me. My brain and body started functioning with the morphine beginning to leave my system, and the Demerol taking over to help the pain.

As I began coming-to, staying quiet while I started to look around the room, a nurse came in and took the chart from the bottom of my bed. After she finished reading, she looked up at me and saw that my eyes were wide open now looking right at her. I don't remember exactly what she said, but she started telling me in a very callus manner that it was time for me to get up and start doing whatever she was telling me to do. Her tone was so rude and nasty there was no way I was going to listen to one more word of what this woman was saying to me. After she was finished, I said, "I don't know who you think you are talking to, but you can leave my room, get the charge nurse, and never step foot back in here." Mike and my mom started laughing saying, "She's back." They may think it's funny that I don't take any negative rude behavior off of anyone, but if you take one awful attitude or comment from one medical person, in my personal experience, you may as well chalk it up that you will be receiving many comments from others to come. Being sick with something people do not understand is no fun. It is infuriating at times.

Recovery from the colon removal took quite a while. When someone has a major surgery, walking is so important, no matter how painful it may be. Gas builds up creating pain. Bowel muscles need stimulation to make sure they start functioning properly again. Going to the bathroom can be a difficult thing if you have a surgery that has nothing to do with your digestive system, let alone the removal of the entire colon. I knew how important it was for me to get up and move around, so I began moving by walking to the bathroom first. The Demerol eased the pain enough to get going. I was very happy they had switched the medication.

Mike told me what had happened the two days prior. No one knew about the fact that I was a Poor Metabolizer for the CYP2D6 allele until November 2012 because none of the doctors I had been seeing in 2008 bothered to tell me. I told everyone how each medication made me feel and it seemed like no one wanted to believe one word I was saying. I felt completely alone, until I found out what was going on physically with my body. I still do not understand how no one would believe what I was saying. Medical or family, why did no one listen?

Imagine how much simpler my life would have been if I was informed I was a Poor Metabolizer in a timely fashion. The diagnosis, Poor Metabolizer, came from a test that was done on January 9, 2008. Four years later, in late 2012, I came across it as I was reading through the medical records that I had ordered. The information about the Poor Metabolism was even circled by the doctor who found it out at Temple University. It was important enough to circle, but the doctor forgot to tell me. That is a huge error. Dr. X received copies of all of this information way back then and didn't catch this information either. He was too busy telling me that everything was in my head to actually read my records.

I was given a prescription for Demerol when it was time to leave the hospital to help with my recovery. The surgery was successful! The colon was removed, with the exception of a small bit to attach the small intestine to, and no colostomy bag! I did leave in a pair of Depends, adult diapers, which I ended up wearing for months during my recovery. I'll take that over what the alternative would have been. We all had a lot to deal with when I came home from the hospital.

I had not been able to eat anymore, prior to the surgery, because the colon would not allow food to go through my body. I could eat again! What an incredible feeling to be able to eat again! Going without food, when your body so desperately needs the nutrition and wants to eat, is exhausting and life threatening. No one with Gastroparesis wants to starve. No one wants to lose weight and become so underweight kids clothes are the only clothes that fit, or specially made clothes. No one with this illness wants to throw up. No one with this illness wants to stop doing everyday routine activities. The body physically does not allow the mobility and physical exertion to do the simplest of household tasks like laundry, dishes or cooking. Tachycardia sets in, physical exhaustion, light headed feelings, nausea and weakness. Many other symptoms begin to occur with the progression of this illness.

While I was so excited to be eating again, I was in diapers, could not leave the house for a few weeks, and I was still not feeling well. Something was not right. I did everything I was supposed to do in my recovery from surgery. I was not a big fast food eater, or preservative eater. People with GP have a difficult time digesting the foods God gave us that grow fresh, let alone things people make with preservatives that destroy the body. Being oversensitive to healthy foods makes preservatives, synthetics, and Genetically

Modified (GMOs) foods wreak havoc on my body. These types of foods destroy a body without health issues.

I went back to Dr. Habibi and told him how I was feeling. From his medical standpoint, I was doing fine. He was the surgeon who did an amazing job helping me to live my life without a bag attached to my body to go to the bathroom. He took care of me and looked out for me from every stand point that he was able to, with regard to his specialty. I needed different types of doctors to help now. He did everything he could, and I appreciate that more than he could ever know.

It was time for Gastroenterologists to find the problems now. It was time for DR. X to help put together the doctors who were going to help me to find out what was going on. Answer the questions, "Why did I lose my colon, and why was not one cell functioning?" I was feeling worse and I just wanted it to stop. It was well past time to find out what was going on. That did not happen.

DR. X continued to tell me it was in my head. He continued to patronize me and tell me I needed psychological help. If I did, it was because of his horrible temperament and verbally abusive manner as a physician. Temple University diagnosed me with Gastroparesis in 2008. I did not find out until 2011, during a hospitalization almost a year after I fired Dr. X, who also agreed to let me go to find another physician because he was unable to help me.

Despite what happened, I was nice to Dr. X. I had someone accompany me to my last appointment just in case of any type of negative situation. When we left that last appointment, my friend was very upset with the doctor for not answering her questions about why I was so sick. Instead he blamed me for getting upset in response to the awful things he said about this illness being "more in my head and my attitude than in my body." On my last appointment, no matter what I told him about how I was feeling, he still held his uneducated opinion that this was in my head. Dr. X should have read the records that were sent to him. This is an outrageous oversight for anyone to have made. I told Dr. X exactly how I was feeling the entire time I had been his patient. As well as the many other doctors who were specialists he referred me to. No one listened, and no one double checked records to see if there was anything that came up that was overlooked. I was just a dollar figure, a patient id, a social security number. I was not a human being who deserved the "Right to Life," like everyone else deserved it seemed.

Dr. X made me feel subhuman on so many occasions. In some ways I felt like he was making it his mission to drill into my husband's head that everything I was feeling was in my head. Dr. X said there was no explanation for what was going on. Tests and blood work were always "fine," "ok." When I requested records and looked at them for myself, many blood tests showed anemia from low red cell counts on multiple occasions, and other parts being counted and tested were marked too low or too high. My white count would not rise for a couple of years to fight infection, and not one infection specialist could explain why.

I had to make things change. Now that I am using certain wellness products, my blood work has leveled out. I am still not feeling well, and my white count still won't come up to fight infection, however, positive changes are still happening. Regardless of what blood work does or doesn't say, and what the tests do or do not say, I will continue to speak out about Gastroparesis, Ehlers-Danlos, Dysautonomia, Mitochondria Syndrome, and so many other illnesses and symptoms that go along with these illnesses, until it is my time to go home to Heaven.

Throughout this book, it is my *hope* that you will be able to walk away with knowledge, understanding, and respect for those who are forced to live with Gastroparesis,Ehlers-Danlos,

Dysautonomia, and other Silent Illnesses. Being a friend and providing support is a tremendous gift you could give. There are so many tasks in a day that most people don't think about, they just do. For those living with Silent Illnesses, there isn't enough energy for a day to begin with, so it is important that we do the most important things and leave the rest until whenever. To have a friend stop by to see how you are feeling, do a load of dishes, throw in a load of laundry, run a vacuum through the house or any other type of help, is a gift that will brighten anyone's day. Someone who just cares because they want to, and no other reason? That is special.

Living without a colon means risk of dehydration all of the time. I was living on IV nutrition prior to the colon being removed, and was able to get off after I was able to bring in foods. I was continuing to feel worse, even though I was now able to go to the bathroom and eat somewhat again, something was still not right. My caloric intake was high enough to sustain me at times. However, I was unable to get the hydration I needed due to the loss of my colon. I kept landing in the emergency room in so much pain that continued under my right rib and throughout my belly, in addition to dehydration and malnutrition bouts. I also was put on IV nutrition again.

My body needed help with hydration and nutrition. Due to my allergies, my body fights itself and anything foreign. Having a life line puts my body at risk, whether a PICC line or Central line; I have developed life threatening blood infections which included multiple bouts with septicemia. I have had to stay in the hospital for days to weeks at a time.

This continued for four more years. I ended up having 5 PICC lines and 5 Central lines from 2007 until 2013. Septicemia and other blood infections are very difficult to fight. I give God all of the glory and praise for carrying me through this life and all of the difficulties it has shown me. I know without my *faith* in God, not religion but *faith*, I would not be sitting here writing this book today. I know that God has always carried me in His arms and there is not one day in my entire life that I do not know God. I am very *blessed* to know His incredible love and strength. I may have lost a colon, but I gained a testimony for His glory.

Life without a colon changed our entire family's lives. There were so many provisions that had to be made. We couldn't go many places, since living without a diaper had not become possible for months after the surgery. I still had to have a nurse come once a week, just as I had prior to the colon removal. I was not able to stay off of the IV nutrition because of the lack of water absorption due to no colon. The colon is where the absorption of water takes place. I still had my energy, still had my muscles, and still able to do many physical things. Even though I had the drive to live, and passion for life, my body was getting weaker and wouldn't let me do everything I could do during the majority of my life. I had learned how to endure not feeling well throughout my life, as things slowly worsened.

My family was not very understanding of the fact that my body was getting weaker. In their eyes, I still looked like the same person. To them, I still acted like the same person, so there was no way I could be feeling as horrible as I was feeling. While I was getting so much weaker, my family did not want to believe that I could no longer do the cleaning, dishes, dinner, and everything else I did around the house and outside of the house. My daughter, who was able to depend on me for the majority of her life, could no longer depend on me. I was just not the same person, and no one could understand. If my own husband and mother would not understand, and there was no one to help, how could my daughter understand all of this? Perhaps we wouldn't have had such a difficult time if I had not been so alone fighting all of this without someone to lean on. I love my daughter more than she can ever know. It seemed the sicker I got, the further she withdrew.

In and out of the hospital, on and off of TPN, as well as eight week stretches of physical therapy and occupational therapy to try to build muscle and save the muscle I had. Each year it becomes increasingly difficult to function. While my life was spared through removing the colon, functioning became a whole new ball game for me. I was used to being Superwoman. I was a single parent for 14 years. When work needed to be done on my car, or other types of work needed to be done, I did it. I was a gymnast when I was young. I carried loads of groceries in from the grocery store in one trip to save multiple trips which meant dragging my daughter the entire time. I could move furniture, go for fast paced walks and enjoy time outside having fun in the sun. I could do so many things before I became too sick and too weak.

I gradually came to a place where any type of normal function was no longer my life. Had the colon not been removed, my risk of another perforation was too high and could have ended my life. Fighting and surviving another bout with septicemia from the intestine was not a risk I was going to take. Fighting an infection like that is very difficult. I am so thankful to have had my colon removed. I wish more was known about Gastroparesis, Ehlers-Danlos, and other illnesses I have to fight so that I, and the millions of others living with Silent Illnesses receive the compassion and care someone with a diagnosis of breast cancer, pancreatic cancer, ALS, or any other serious illness would receive. Illnesses which cause death should not be in competition for attention and funding. Gastroparesis and other Silent Illnesses are extremely painful, debilitating many to the point of needing physical assistance to function, and just as serious deserving the attention many other debilitating illnesses receive.

###

Romans 8:18-20

For I consider [from the standpoint of faith] that the sufferings of the present life are not worthy to be compared with the glory that is about to be revealed to us and in us! For [even the whole] creation [all nature] waits eagerly for the children of God to be revealed. For the creation was subjected to frustration and futility, not willingly [because of some intentional fault on its part], but by the will of Him who subjected it...

Chapter 4

The Beginning of the End

On May 25, 2011, my 44th birthday, I woke up, looked around my room, and said, "I will not die this way!" I vowed to never be admitted to the hospital again. I had decided all tests from now until I was dead, would be done outpatient. I couldn't worry anymore about doctors or nurses thinking I should be in the emergency room, or admitted to the hospital. I was so tired of being told to go to the emergency room, and have the doctors and nurses in the emergency room treat me like I am a drug seeker. That word alone is a scary word after everything I have had to experience. Situations that I could not possibly have imagined actually existed.

I am not the only one who has experienced what I am sharing with you. For so many, the health care that we receive is less than adequate. I had to fight for my life in 2008, and again multiple times after that. I am still living a health nightmare which I choose to take one moment at a time. I choose to advocate for myself, and stand up for what I know to be the truth of what is going on in my body. Dr. X told me everything was in my head and that I was depressed. I told him I was not. I told him I was aggravated because no one was listening or trying to figure out what was going on, but I was 100% not depressed. I was researching and developing Teen Moms Fresh Start, I was writing, and I was researching my own symptoms to see if I could figure out what was going on.

Depression is the diagnosis so many doctors like to throw around when they cannot figure out what is wrong with a person. Physicians "practice medicine" on people who come to them for help. No human being on this earth knows how to fix everything that is happening to our bodies; so, physicians "practice" what they learn in a school setting, on people who I choose to call "clients" for this example. The medical profession prefers the term "patients."

When we go to the doctor or any other type of medical facility, we pay for a service. A medical service to answer questions we have about ourselves and what we are feeling. When we have questions about what we are feeling, questions about something that is keeping us from living the best life we can, we pay money to discuss our situation. We pay physicians for their services in aiding us to find out what is happening to our bodies. We pay for their time. People have come to depend on doctors for all of their answers as opposed to depending on themselves. It seems too many people want the quick fix pills that lead to worse problems down the road.

As individuals, we absolutely know what we are feeling. The turn-around time that doctors try to stick to does not work for those with chronic and terminal illnesses. Regardless of how much time you take with the physician you are working with, when you know there is something going on, try to create a plan of action that you and your doctor will follow. People seeking medical answers and support forget that we are the ones most important in the patient/physician relationship. We need answers to questions about our health that affects our ability to live. Not scapegoat diagnoses like depression and anxiety.

The answers lie more in our own knowledge than with doctors. Doctors are people who went to school. They are not God, not above the law, and not above you or me. We are all people, all important, and all deserving proper respect and attention. When we have a problem, a health issue, we should be making notes of what is happening in writing, and have those notes placed in our files along with the doctors' notes. From everything that I have been through, I see many doctors who just do not listen to their clients. I was told in February, 2012, by a Gastroenterology Specialist at Hopkins, that he did not see Gastroparesis from a Gastric Emptying Scan performed a couple of years prior, so I was not suffering like I was explaining. He did, however, think I had Fibromyalgia, and gave me a script to see his Rheumatologist within 48 hours. I was so sick and in so much pain with the digestive system and all related pain I was there for, I just wanted help. Help that would not come for a very long time. The digestive issues were the reason I scheduled the appointment. Not to be told to see a Rheumatologist for pain. I wanted help for my belly, which I did not receive, but the doctor was paid anyway. I cannot begin to imagine the numbers of appointments I have paid for in my lifetime, only to be told to go see someone else for one reason or another, that had nothing to do with what was happening to my digestive system.

I had let this doctor know I've already been diagnosed with Gastroparesis and informed him of all of the other tests I had done since that particular test he was reading. The test he had was done not long after the removal of my colon in 2008. I met with him in 2012. The test he was looking at could have never ruled out or diagnosed Gastroparesis because of when they did the test and the conditions under which the test was done. I was diagnosed well before that test had been done, and confirmed through other tests after the colon was removed. The doctor wouldn't listen, he didn't want to follow up for the reason I was there to begin with, and there was no plan of action with regard to my health and what I was going to do next.

I did not go back to see him after that experience. He showed me that there was no way that we could work together by refusing to discuss the issues that I wanted to discuss. Tests done after the Gastric Emptying Scan that this doctor was only referring to, showed Gastroparesis, esophageal problems, but was then quickly dismissed. From where I'm standing, what I saw was a doctor who spent the 15 minute time period and then had no more time for me. Time's up. Move on to the next patient. His only recommendation was his Rheumatologist referral.

The particular doctor who wanted me to see the Rheumatologist right away was one I had attempted to see on two separate occasions. Four years apart in visits hoping things had changed. I gave him a second chance hoping for a better outcome. The outcome was the same so there was no sense in wasting any more of my time or money. When I was a single parent, and had the responsibility of owning a business to make ends meet, not one time was I reimbursed for the outrageous amount of time I have lost from my life.

No amount of money can ever reimburse the time taken away from my daughter and the stress created by the physicians who told me everything I was dealing with was in my head. My daughter and I were the ones who had to live with the excruciating pain of my colon dying, and all of the nausea, vomiting, diarrhea, constipation, bloody stools, and crippling pain I had to live. The medical community wants to be paid when you don't show up, but they don't want to pay you for the hours, months and years of wasted time they cause. They don't want to see you if you are more than 15 minutes late, expect payment for time when appointments are missed, and keep us waiting because of overbooking.

Our time is every bit as important as a doctor's time. We are all human. We all do different things. The people who collect our trash are equally as important as doctors. How could anyone run a business with trash piled up in their offices or hospitals? Unless we all respect each other, not the job title, the problems we face within the medical profession, and within our communities in general, will continue. We will never have the peace and support we all need to get through this life.

Too many people sit high on their pedestals and point fingers, but will generally not want to accept responsibility for their mistakes. They have no problem accepting recognition for their accomplishments, and all the while human beings lives are affected. Doctors are human and make as many mistakes as any other human beings on the planet. Please advocate for yourself. The medical definition of Gastroparesis means paralysis of the gastric system. Gastric means stomach in medical terms. The true definition is much more complicated than that. I *hope* that I am able to paint a clear picture for you about the severity of this illness. I *hope* to successfully express the absolute need to be supportive of anyone who is living with this illness, as with anyone living with any other chronic or life threatening illness or disease.

I have been sick with digestive issues as far back as I can remember, and before. When my daughter was about 7 years old, I was so sick to the point I had to lay on the floor of the bathroom, with my head on the floor just outside of the bathroom in the hallway on the carpet for some cushion. My daughter sat stroking my hair because I could not move or breathe normally from the pain. Living with chronic nausea, intense pain, and throwing up regularly because my body does not want food, is no "walk in the park." Being forced to live in a 10 plus degree pain that does not go away, only reducing by a couple of points in between bouts, is like being tortured in a body prison that no one will give you the key to. My daughter was severely affected by all that I had to live through because no one wanted to listen.

The past 6 years have been the hardest, because of having to fight to stay alive. When I was very young, into my teens, my grandmother would have me go out back and pick mint when I would complain of my stomach. She also used to say to me, "If you say your stomach hurts, it's going to hurt." My mother doesn't remember me doubling over in pain when I was little. I sure remember. How can anyone forget something that hurts that bad without relief in sight? I spent quite a bit more time with my grandparents, including living with them on and off for a huge part of my life growing up. Perhaps that is why my grandmom could remember, and my mom couldn't. My mom was trying to raise three children by herself, from the time I was five years old. My grandmother was the one who seemed to think I just had a belly ache and complaining. I'll never know how different my life could have been if someone would have just listened a long time ago. It was very frustrating to have to feel that terrible, tell everyone how I felt, and have no one listen.

The frustration grew as time went on as I became an adult. When I was about 19, I began going to doctors to find out what was wrong with me. During my adult life, doctors did so many tests without conclusive results for anything but Irritable Bowel, an ulcer, Diverticulosis, Ulcerative Colitis, sensitivities to dairy and gluten, patches on the lining of my intestines that were flaring up with allergic reactions to foods, and who knows what else I was told. It is hard to remember everything. The proper tests were not prescribed to detect GP until I was 41 years old, and went out of state to Temple University in Philadelphia.

As awful as I was feeling, I do not understand why the motility tests were never performed until just before I lost my colon 5 years ago. I am now 46 years old, and have had to endure a lifetime of digestive issues that debilitated my life in multiple ways. The first time I filed for Disability to help while I was trying to find out what was going on, was about 15 years ago. I filed approximately 6 times from 15 years ago, until about 5 years ago. I have been living with this, undiagnosed, my entire life. I have pushed, as so many others do, feeling miserable but going on anyway. There is no other choice but to continue on. To lie down and just give in to this can mean your death. There are different severities of this illness. Some are mild, some are moderate, and some are severe. No two people are identical, no matter how similar in symptoms they are. People tolerate different foods and can be allergic to different things.

December of 2011, I prayed for God to take me home. I could not bear to go on another moment. I had come down with one of the worst flus that had been going around that winter. My granddaughter brought it home from a daycare she had begun attending. I refused to go in the hospital again. Mike had already left for work when the fever spiked and I became bed ridden. I was using a walker to get from my bed to the bathroom as well. I called Mike to turn around and come back home. My granddaughter, Carissa, was home. I was so sick I could not get out of the bed, and needed someone to be in the house with Carissa to help with what she needed, and for me, just in case of anything. I remember my granddaughter wanting me to get up and play with her. I just quietly talked to her until Mike came home. Mike took care of Carissa, and kept checking on me to see if I needed anything. What he didn't understand was how sick I really was. He didn't understand that I had no more fight left. He didn't understand I did not get out of the bed to go to the bathroom or eat because my body was done. I wanted to go home to Heaven.

By the late afternoon, while Mike and Carissa were downstairs, my breathing had gotten to a point where I was only able to take a breath in, exhale, and wait until my body had enough energy to take another breath. I prayed for God to take me home. I prayed so hard for Him to end this chamber of torture I was being forced to live in. I asked to come home so that I did not have to feel like this anymore. I wanted to feel peace, warmth, and love. I could not even open my eyes anymore.

While I was praying, I could feel the tears fall down the sides of my face. I wanted to come Home. God told me it was not my time. There was still too much to do. I knew I had to stay. I told God I needed more of His strength. I needed the strength to get up out of the bed, stay out of the hospital, and do everything I had been working so hard to accomplish. I asked God to fill me with all of His strength, surround me with all of His angels to protect me from this awful illness, and get me to my feet so I could make a difference.

If I died, my daughter would have been on this earth alone. After I remarried, the family days she and I always had, began to disappear. I married a family that was not close. Not like Sam and I were. They didn't talk very much to one another, not the way Sam and I did. Our way of life was much different than there's. Sam and I were used to snuggling, hugging, holding hands, laughing, crying, and all of the other incredibly wonderful things families do together. Mike and his children weren't as expressive, which isn't a bad thing, as long as you can still communicate effectively. Please do not be afraid to talk to your family and friends. Tell people how you really feel, so that people can learn to live together. We are all different, but we all have similarities as well. It would be so nice if people could just accept the differences, without having to go through so much judgment and so many problems along the way.

People need to learn to stop judging one another. Don't assume you know why a person is going through difficult times. Listen to what others have to say and understand that everyone goes through trials. Some live more difficult lives than others. It would be nice to see people reaching out and asking their neighbors if there is anything they need, instead of judging why things are the way they are, not the way they think they should be. I miss the old days when I could walk across the street and borrow sugar, milk, or eggs, and vice versa. It was a completely different time period.

I would not wish for anyone to go through the difficulties we have had with blending two families. At this point, we have not been successful. While on this earth, it is so important that we work in collaboration with one another. We are merely pieces of a puzzle, and the puzzle is not complete if the pieces do not fit together properly because of a lack of connection. Each of us is a piece of the puzzle of life. If we do not stand by one another, many fall, and the puzzle always remains incomplete.

Luke 10:27

And he replied, "You shall love the Lord your God with all your heart, and with all your soul,

and with all your strength, and with all your mind;
and your neighbor as yourself."

Chapter 5

It Begins Again, the Diagnosis

That May 11th, when I said I was not going to be admitted to the hospital anymore, I meant it. But a couple of months later, I began being admitted for twelve to fourteen day stretches at a time, as opposed to two to seven day stretches. My white cell count had not come up for a couple of years, which made any kind of illness or even a cold difficult to fight. During a hospital stay at Howard County General, one of the Infection Specialists came in to talk to me about my white blood cell not increasing to fight infection, and that he did not understand why. I was dealing with life threatening blood infections from the IV line for my nutrition that I desperately needed to live. I wanted to know what tests could be done to find out why my white cell count would not rise to fight infection anymore. I wanted to know what could be done to find out why I couldn't eat and had to live off IV nutrition. I wanted to know why I was so sick and in so much pain.

The doctor did not know what to test for. It didn't seem like anyone knew what to test for. Test after test, year after year, no answers. I just could not understand any of this. Somehow all of these people performing or reading all of these tests said everything was fine, or a mild this or a mild that. How could that be? The problem was not in my head, as everyone had suggested for years, it was in my body. So what could be done? I wanted answers and was getting nowhere.

I wondered if I was the only one this sick, since doctors could not figure out what was happening. I ended up being transferred to Georgetown University in DC during one of the stays with Howard County General. It was a horrible transfer. An extremely difficult and frustrating wait to be admitted. I was told I was going to be transferred into the hospital, not the emergency room. They transferred me by ambulance from an admitted patient at Howard County General Hospital to sit in the emergency room of Georgetown University to wait to be assessed through triage. How in the world did this happen? How was I not transferred to the hospital itself, to specialists at this hospital since Howard County was unable to help me? According to Howard County, they did not have the expertise to help me. There was no communication by doctors from one hospital to another. Howard County General Hospital just let me go as if I was never there. None of the records were sent with me when I was transferred. No information about the white count not rising and their inability to find out the problem. Nothing. I went through another horrific emergency room visit when I was entirely too sick and I ended up having to spend the entire night before they finally admitted me to the floor.

If I were in the public eye in anyway, the negative situations would have never occurred.

After experiencing the difference in treatment when someone I know who is in the public eye came in one day to my emergency room, I was appalled. I was just some patient being judged and treated horribly, until he walked in my room. After that, when the people who were working at the Howard County General Hospital ER changed from being horrible to treating me as if I owned the world. I was furious. I was furious to see how different people are treated depending on status. The way I see it, if I were the president, an actor or actress, someone in the public eye with money, I would have never been accused of being a drug seeker or talked to like I am an idiot without an ounce of understanding. Who knows, if I were in the public eye, perhaps we would have a cure by now.

Why so many doctors think I, or anyone else, want to be sick in an emergency room or hospital, faking pain from the problems from the Gastroparesis and the Ehlers-Danlos just to get drugs is actually a ridiculous judgment. While there are people who are addicted to prescription drugs, and have pain in the belly from withdraw, this is not the type of pain someone with Gastroparesis goes through. Imagine always living with areas that feel like they are going to rupture on a regular basis. Many of the drugs they prescribe do increase constipation. While I had to go through years of trying different medications to find something I was not allergic too, I found that some of the pain meds increased the constipation, while the Demerol that I am not allergic to, did not and still has not increased constipation. I have had to take Demerol over the past year. Constipation from this medication has never been an issue.

While I was in Georgetown University Hospital, it was then that I found out the name, Gastroparesis. Finally, an answer. I asked the doctors how they found out. I was told that they requested the records from Temple University and the diagnosis was there. This is where I say,

"WHAT?" I find out in 2011, from Georgetown University, who pulled records from 2008. My life became impossible to live. I could not stay out of the hospital. I could not stop throwing up, which I had to have Botox injections inside of my stomach at the pyloric sphincter area to stop the vomiting. In the stomach, Botox lasts approximately 3 to 4 months, not the 6 months that it lasts on superficial skin like the face. There is much more movement in the stomach, as well as a different environment than the face, therefore making the Botox wear off quicker.

When I first heard the diagnosis, Gastroparesis, I thought this must be something rare for them to overlook for so many years and accuse me over being a drug seeker. I did have to hire a psychiatrist and drug addiction counselor to document everything that was happening each week in the medical profession to protect me from what was happening. I would not touch any narcotics, with the exception of Demerol, because

I know that the other drugs can cause horrible reactions, and could end my life. If I am this huge drug seeker, than why would I not take anything else that they tried to give me? They tried to give me every narcotic under the sun, except for Demerol. I find that to be neglectful, abusive, stereotyping, and prejudiced to treat me so harshly. I have had doctors say things like, "You will lay there in all of that pain instead of take a different medication?" I have to always repeat myself and tell them I cannot take anything else, if I do, I risk my own life and I refuse to do it anymore. I will not let doctors try meds on me to see if I have a reaction for themselves.

I used to let them order a small dose of a medication I cannot tolerate to prove I couldn't take it through the reactions I would have. I refuse to do that to myself anymore just because a doctor wants to stereotype me. This is no different than any form of racism. In fact, it is worse because the medications can stop a life immediately without any discussion. Racism reaps hatred, and death in circumstances can be a possibility, but most of the time not an immediate death that a drug could cause.

After I left the hospital, I was not going to be diagnosed with something that I knew nothing about, so I began to research. I had to find out what was going on. I wanted to get better. I didn't want to keep getting worse. Through research, I found that there are millions who are living with these illnesses. I found an incredible Geneticist, Clair Francomano, M.D., who diagnosed me with Ehlers-Danlos, which may be the overlying culprit of GP. She also diagnosed me with Dysautonomia and Mast Cell Activation Disorder. The drug seeker judgment continues, even though I cannot take anything but Demerol. I continue to search for a general doctor who will be willing to work with me and all of these illnesses. All of the personal physicians to date say they do not know enough about these illnesses and suggest I find a doctor who is more knowledgeable or specializes in Ehlers-Danlos or Gastroparesis. Dr. Francomano, my geneticist, is the only doctor in all of these decades to give me such an enormous amount of respect, along with being considerate while diagnosing what is happening to me. Too many doctors immediately said I was depressed, wrote prescriptions and quickly got through my visits to bring in the next patient. An assembly line of patients. Each time I would leave the doctors' offices, I left without answers. I was so tired of being told I was depressed. When I would get angry for being told I am depressed, many of those doctors would say anger is a sign of depression. In return, I would say, "I'm not depressed, I'm furious you are not listening." I cannot wait to finally find a physician who wants to learn more to be able to help others as well.

I went through so many phases of being mad and hurt after so many years of being told there was nothing wrong with me. Being told this was in my head, while it is in my guts. When I was diagnosed at Temple University, the doctor put in the first few visits that he was not sure if this was psychological or not. Tests confirmed I had Colonic Inertia and Gastroparesis, but they decided not to tell me about the Gastroparesis. Perhaps I could have had an easier time living with this, had I known early on.

My life was extremely difficult in so many ways. Raising my beautiful little girl on my own, as sick as I was, became the norm. I never gave up. I tried so hard to do as much as possible and not let it negatively affect my daughter's life. We were so active when she was born throughout elementary school, but the degree of difficulty became too much by the time she entered middle school. We can do our best to not let our negative situations affect our children, but the truth is, no matter how hard we try, our children see what is happening. If you are the only one everyone is depending on, it is absolutely impossible to hide it all of the time. The bouts of pain that drop you to your knees on the floor, or in a ball in bed, no one can hide. The overwhelming nausea, vomiting, weakness, and other stressful symptoms that are impossible to hide. While my colon was steadily dying, and yes, I could feel it, I was told the physical problems were in my head and could not get disability. It was easier for me to work for myself than other people, so I did. I worked with a couple different companies during the first decade of Sam's life, but in the end, I would end up sicker than when I started. Working for myself was the best option.

After I found out about the diagnosis during the George Washington University admission, I started researching. I was astounded by the amount of information available to the public, as well as the lack of effort to do something to help so many people suffering and struggling to live. In August of 2003, a White Paper entitled, "Gastroparesis and Related Digestive Motility

Diseases, a Medical Crisis" prepared by Gastroparesis and Dysmotilities Association, was submitted to NIH, Congress, and Senate. Here we are, an entire decade later, and no more has been done by these political bodies to pass legislation and protocols on a federal and state level. Too many people have died since the 2003 paper calling for our government to wake up and take responsibility for what is happening in our country.

I could not sit around and not do anything, so I decided to create a website, Gastroparesis and ME, and share all of the information that I came upon through research. I wanted everyone to know what is happening out here so that we can find the support we need to make life better for all of us. Through research and Dr. Francomano entering my life as my geneticist, I have found that Ehlers-Danlos (EDS) to be the huge culprit for my Gastroparesis (GP). Many with GP have been diagnosed with EDS, and vice versa, but many more have never heard of it. That is something that will change in time, as long as we continue to educate the public about everything that is happening in our country in the medical world.

###

Matthew 7:1-2

Do not judge and criticize and condemn [others unfairly with an attitude of self-righteous superiority as though assuming the office of a judge], so that you will not be judged [unfairly]. For just as you [hypocritically] judge others [when you are sinful and unrepentant], so will you be judged; and in accordance with your standard of measure [used to pass out judgment], judgment will be measured to you.

Chapter 6

Family Devastation

Since my first difficult fight to stay alive in the beginning of 2008, my family took a horrible blow. Septicemia was the first gram positive blood infection, among many more to come. This particular bout with septicemia came from the bacteria from the feces that had gotten into my blood stream. This was caused by a colon perforation that was due to the Colonic Inertia and Ehlers-Danlos. The Colonic Inertia, and the rest of the digestive tract paralysis problems, I learned were due to Ehlers-Danlos. Mike and Sam were there every day and were so afraid they were going to lose me. Mike stuck by my side while taking care of Sam who was only 15 at the time.

This has affected my family in so many ways. My daughter has been affected the most and had the most to lose. From the time my daughter was conceived, I knew she was a girl. I knew her name would be Sam as far back as I could remember. No matter what the doctor told me quite some time ago, that I would probably never become pregnant again because of the destruction from the Endometriosis, I always knew I would have a girl and her name would be Sam. She is my miracle baby and doesn't know just how much of a miracle she is. I thank God for gifting me with such a wonderful person to love and raise. I'm just so sorry that I could not find out what was wrong earlier to have the support I needed throughout my life, as well as her life. Everyone, including my family, did not believe I was as sick as I was. *If I could push my own wheelchair, I couldn't be that sick,* was their mentality, as well as an actual comment that was made. Their mentality should have been how great it was that no matter how bad I was feeling, I didn't want to sit in the wheelchair and give up so young. I fought constantly to feel better and not give in to becoming bedridden or housebound. I wanted to be active and live.

My daughter's smile could light an entire room. When my daughter was born, through her entire childhood, and as she grew, she was so breathtakingly beautiful and so kind hearted. I remember this one day she wanted to play with a toy her friend had left over our house. She refused to touch it without calling and getting permission from her friend. She was between the ages of six and seven at that time. I carry a business card around that she wrote on the back of: "10/21/02 -- I love my mom so much that I could explode. She is my only mommy in the world. She taught everything I know and that's why I am the way I am, caring."

Now here we are, 11 years later, and our relationship has drifted apart to almost nothing. I miss my daughter more than words can say. She has distanced herself for many reasons. I do believe, if I had not ended up sick the way I have been, incapable of doing so many things I could do when she was younger, our relationship would not have drifted. We would have had a lifetime of time together.

My energy is like a stream that runs dry. I may start out my days with a small amount of energy, but, as the moments go by, my energy becomes depleted with any amount of exertion. I am very weak, even though I don't look it most of the time, which creates the inability to do so many physical things I used to do. Since I don't look like I feel, perhaps in Sam's eyes, she thinks I don't want to do anything with her. I don't really know. I truly wish our family would have had support. My family is not the only family to deal with stress from chronic illness and not have the support to work through it. As with other chronic to terminal illnesses, there should be counseling for the family to help them through the stressors that come along with illness.

Samantha respected people at a very young age. I have always respected people for who they are, their differences, as well as similarities. God created each one of us unique. She was such an amazing person from the time she was born.

The sicker I became, the harder Sam's world became. My first hospitalization left me in the bed at Mike's house to recover when she was fifteen years old. Sam was just beginning her young life. Moving her to a different school seemed wrong at the time, when in hind sight, it would have been the better choice. Life is a journey. We make many decisions that may not be the best decisions, but seems like the best one at the time. I mention this because none of us will ever do everything perfect no matter how hard we strive to. Judging another person is nothing but a waste of time. Nothing is perfect but God. There is only one perfection and we are not it. I wish I had more caring people physically in my life to help get through some of the most incredibly difficult and debilitating circumstances I have ever been through. If it were not for my *faith*, my relationship with God, I know that I would not have been able to survive this otherwise.

Sam and I had to depend on my uncle for support in 2006. That was the year prior to my first IV nutrition line and constant hospitalizations. In 2006, I had my right ovary out. The last of my female organs destroyed by Endometriosis. I was really not feeling well and I was still being told everything was fine. Blood work fine, tests fine, everything was always fine. That same year, I ended up with pneumonia, pleurisy, and a fractured rib, which landed me in the emergency room of Mercy Hospital, in Baltimore. They sent me into a steroidal psychosis by injecting me with IV steroids, when I can barely tolerate oral steroids. I was already on a low dose of Prednisone that was already creating agitation at that point.

I don't even remember receiving the injection of steroids I was given. I react to just about everything it seems so far. That was not an enjoyable experience. Being in a psychosis is so strange. I could remember things, but I could not communicate to anyone to let them know that I was afraid and needed to go home. I was not being taken care of during that hospital visit. I wasn't shocked, but I wasn't up for the stress. After nine days, I could communicate again and insisted Dr. X take care of me from home. I was released that day. Dr. X ordered a bone scan which determined I had a fractured rib, on top of the pneumonia and pleurisy discovered on the emergency room x-ray. That was the first time I landed in bed at home needing so much care.

Being as sick as I was and having to move in with Mike to get the at home care I needed, I was afraid to switch Sam to a new school would prove worse for Sam, not better. Not a wise decision. My uncle did not have the ability to handle authority.

Quite a bit more went on when my daughter was with my uncle than I knew about. All of the rules we lived by seemed to fly out the window. It was getting more difficult for me to stand on my own two feet and keep our rules in place. Moving in with Mike, and living with a family who had an entirely different structure than we were used to, was an extremely difficult move on all of us. An adjustment that did not work very well for anyone. Going from rules to almost no rules, during a crucial time in my daughter's life, was probably the worst thing I could have ever done. I didn't realize what we would have to give up.

At that point in time, I needed more help than I had ever needed in my life. With all of my heart, I believed Mike loved me with all of his heart. He still brought me flowers. He still came up to see how I was and would sit and talk with me. I had never hit the bed the way I did from that bout of pneumonia. I could not bounce back. I'm sure that's because the colon was not functioning and I was not getting the nutrition and hydration that I needed to maintain homeostasis. The colon was removed about a year and a half after the pneumonia hospitalization.

I know Sam feels like I abandoned her. I didn't. So many times I have felt like I abandoned her. I didn't. I was doing my best. My body was sick and I was doing everything I could to function without the proper medical care for my health. When I landed in Mercy Hospital emergency room with pneumonia, it was the beginning of a steady decline that we all had to deal with. Dr. X was supposed to set things up so that I was a direct admit. I saw him the day I went into the emergency room. He had recommended hospitalization. My daughter and I looked at each other when Dr. X suggested this. We agreed, because of the seriousness of my breathing situation, being admitted was probably the best thing to protect me. Looking back, what a mistake that was.

A mistake to trust that this doctor had my best interest at heart. A mistake that had horrible ramifications on my daughter's and my relationship. The emergency room staff dosed me too high with steroids, which sent me soaring into a psychosis. I was talking about kittens and other things when I was trying to tell my family to get me out of the hospital. I was afraid. I tried to tell them I was being mistreated, and everyone working was staring at me passing me by, as opposed to helping. I did not have one test while I was in there for a nine day period. At one point I remember screaming at Mike, Sam, and my mom, to get out because they were playing charades trying to guess what I was saying. I know Sam's feelings were hurt the worst. Her strong mom who had handled everything was reduced to nothing. Living sick like this has taken so much away from my daughter and I. I miss that girl.

My body cannot tolerate steroids and I had already begun a Prednisone steroid taper. The emergency room staff did not bother to see if I was sensitive to steroids before they dosed me with more steroids. I was very afraid at that hospital. They were not taking care of me, and to top it all off, I couldn't communicate to tell anyone. I needed to be cared for from home where I had access to my nebulizer and medicines when I needed them, as opposed to when the nurses were able to get to me. At home, I wouldn't be alone and at that point in time, my family was there to look out for me.

The nurses would watch me stare off into space, through hallucination trips I have never been on before, and they would laugh. Between the steroids, and all of the other meds, I was off in another world on a number of occasions during the first half or more of the stay.

One night, when no one was there with me at the hospital, I drifted off into a hallucination. If I had to deal with a hallucination, I was so happy that it was with my daughter. I really thought I was sitting with Sam on a green grassy hill. The sun was shining bright, with one beautiful, full, green tree to our left and we were having the best time. We were laughing, eating ice cream cones and talking. We always talked. We loved talking prior to me getting so sick. We would sit and snuggle and talk or read a book. Sometimes we would snuggle to watch one of her favorite movies. My daughter and I were inseparable. I remember every smile, every stroke of her beautiful hair, every laugh, every time she told me how much she loved me, and every time I told her I loved her more than all the skies and all the trees. My daughter and I had such an incredible relationship that I miss so much. I used to be Superwoman, now I can barely move my own weight around, which isn't much. I was my daughter's rock. Her father was never someone to be depended on, or trusted. We had my uncle to depend on, but he had many disabilities of his own. On New Year's Eve, December 31, 2010, my uncle passed from a massive heart attack. RIP Uncle Tim!! Thank you for all you did for us!!

My uncle was the best!! Uncle Tim loved us very much. I grew up with my uncle. He was a very big part of my life. We worked on cars together. I loved to go free-riding in his cars with him. In the Jeep, we would climb hills and go for distance rides through land in VA. I grew up going camping with my uncle, along with the first and only wife he ever had, their two sons (my cousins), and his wife's family. When my aunt and uncle divorced, it was as if the entire families divorced. I didn't want that. I was so close to both of them, as well as the family on my aunt's side. Sometimes people who you think are family, end up not being who you thought they were. I have had that happen and cannot understand how people can do that. I have seen it happen to so many other people as well.

While I have fought to keep this body going, I have tried my best to live. I landed in the hospital on too many occasions. My uncle did all he could for my daughter and I. Some family members did a lot to criticize. They were not as supportive during this time period. We did the best we could under the circumstances I was living under, but most family never believed I was as sick as I was. Many judgmental comments were made throughout the years. It sucks when people judge you for how you handle a difficult situation. How does anyone really know what choices they would make, until they are actually faced with a situation? It is God's place to judge, not ours.

It is amazing how harsh people can be to people who are sick. It would be a perfect world if everyone could see how their own actions or words affect people. None of us are perfect. Each person plays a role and does have responsibility in most problems or situations that arise between people. As human beings, we need to be willing to look at ourselves and accept those responsibilities. To continue to place blame in the lap of others, keeps the vicious cycle of insanity going. Negativity hurts. To be able to look at ourselves and realize we can do something different in any situation, gives us the power to be the best we can be without feeling the need to be right about everything. People living with debilitating, deteriorating, and overall difficult illnesses should avoid stressful situations with others or their symptoms could be exacerbated.

Mike and I had a great deal of fun and laughs until I became too sick to do most things. We were out one night, about six years after we had met, and someone had asked us how long we had been together. When we told them six years, they told us they could not believe that two people could still be as in love with each other as we were. I have not loved someone with trust the way I loved Mike. If someone would have told me at any point in this relationship, prior to me becoming disabled, that Mike would not be supportive if I became sick, I would have had to say they were wrong and had no idea what they were talking about. I thought that because of our love, we would make it through life's difficulties. That just didn't happen.

We are still together, almost six years after the removal of my colon, however, our life and marriage is not what I thought it would be. Mike has heart issues, and five stents. If anything would happen to him where he would be unable to work, and I was the one who had the strength, there is nothing I would not do for him. I have taken care of many people in my family. I have not turned my back on anyone who was sick and needed help. I was my grandmom's primary caregiver for a year and a half prior to her passing. A 24-hour, 7-days-a-week responsibility. After my grandfather passed in December of 1991, everyone in the family stepped up and helped my grandmom in any way we could. During the last year and a half of my grandmom's life, she went through so many different changes. I know my grandmom had EDS, chronic constipation and other GI problems, heart attacks, strokes, rupturing vessels, to name some of her health problems. There was limited support and limited resources. After applying as my grandmom's caregiver, it was approximately 13 or 14 months before I ended up being paid by the state to take care of my grandmom. There are caregiver programs on the state level, which is the program I applied for. I had to wait for funds to become available from the specific program she qualified for. There was no way for me to take care of my grandmom day and night, take care of my middle school age daughter, take care of my own body that was doing what it could to take me down, and try to work. I could barely keep up without a break, but through God's Grace I did it. There was no one who could take my place.

My own body was undertaking too much with the progression of my grandmom's health. Instead of medical help for me, I was told by doctors it was in my head and I was depressed. I wish I could make that "D" word disappear. I wasn't depressed, I was exhausted and needed support with my grandmom and daughter, as well as someone in the medical profession who had knowledge of the symptoms I was having to be able to help me. I lived with health issues every day. Nausea, vomiting, pain and weakness for years prior to finding out what was going on. My health was so out of control, it dictated what I could and couldn't do each day. I always over did it because everyone needed so much. I always ended up in tremendous pain, throwing up, gagging, without the support I needed from family, friends, or the medical profession.

About two months after my colon was removed, and for two and a half years after, Mike told me everything was in my head. Not at first though. He let his sister know, during a telephone conversation after my colon was removed, that things would be as normal as normal could be. He let her know that there was a lot of recovery time and we wouldn't really know how life would be until then.

It was only a couple of months after that telephone conversation with his sister that Mike started the "everything was in my head" thing. The initial trigger was Dr. X insisting everything was in my head. He insisted I was so horribly depressed, that I had caused my body to be this sick, I had my colon removed. He also said if I was not committed to a psychiatric facility, my health problems would get worse than they already were. Not long after the stress with Dr. X began, our family began to break down. Mike's daughter started with unrealistic demands about her wedding. My daughter and her husband were having problems that spilled over into our lives. On top of everything, during my stepdaughter's wedding, I had to deal with actions that were completely inappropriate and uncalled for from Mike's ex-wife, and her family. The stress and shock to my body, from all of these situations, increased the problems I was having with my health.

On top of being sick with health problems no one understood, I began living a life of almost complete alienation and isolation. My only way out of the nightmare was to write my way out, while trying to find out what was wrong with me. I didn't know what to do or who to turn to, so I began researching symptoms and illnesses. Reading and writing became my world. I wrote about all types of information that may prove helpful later, thoughts and ideas, as well as poems, blogs not posted yet, and the words on the pages of this book. Writing helped me be strong by giving me a voice when I didn't think I could go on anymore. Even though no one else was hearing my voice at that time, I still felt like writing opened a window so that I could breathe.

It was not until my admission to Georgetown University, in 2011, two and a half years after my colon was removed, that Mike finally broke down and apologized for the hell he had put me through by not listening to me. Even though he broke down, being compassionate and being my partner did not last very long. My daughter had completely pulled away from me by then, and was not very nice to me at that point. Mike's kids never came over after the wedding. There were too many damaging factors, but Mike refused to bring the family together to talk about things so our life as a family could work toward being repaired. Instead, everything continued to simmer and get worse, rather than work together. When one parent gets sick, the entire household is disrupted. But if one parent gets sick, and the family is not understanding, not supportive, and not willing to work together, the beginning of a growing nightmare is formed.

In 2013, Dr. Clair Francomano diagnosed me with Ehlers-Danlos, and suspected that I also had Mast Cell Activation Disorder, and

Dysautonomia. To have actual diagnoses was an incredible breakthrough in my life. This explained so much of what was happening to me. This was also not the first time I was supposed to have seen Dr. Francomano. During one of my admissions to GBMC, in 2011, I was told by one of the doctors, that I would be having genetic testing done while I was in the hospital. The geneticist I would have seen at that time was Dr. Clair Francomano. Instead, one of the GI physicians came in and told me that I would do better in another medical setting. Not only was I being treated like a drug seeker again, I was being kicked out of the hospital as well. With Demerol being the only pain medication my system can handle, being accused of being a drug seeker is absolutely absurd. The doctors constantly try to give me other drugs, but I refuse them and always explain why. Since Demerol is the only pain medication I can take without allergic reactions or over sensitivities, I refuse all other pain medications.

How does this make me a drug seeker? Do I deserve to be kicked out of the hospital because of an opinion, not fact?

What so many of us living with Gastroparesis and related illnesses have to go through to get the help we need is absolutely absurd. Quite often, I have been subjected to inhumane treatment by those in the medical profession, both inpatient in the hospital, and outpatient in the doctors' offices. It is so important that our family and friends are there for us every step of the way. Without their protection, the medical community can get away with anything; whether it is in the best interest of the patient or not. I know from personal experience, and from listening to others who have Gastroparesis and related illnesses. Doctors are people too, and human beings make mistakes. To entertain the thought that a doctor's position makes them better than you or I, or more important, is a huge mistake. Titles do not lift people above being human.

I look back and do not know how, other than by the grace of God, I made it through all of that. I can sit here and tell you how horrible it is to have your doctor tell you all of your health problems are in your head, but it is impossible to understand unless you have been through it. On top of the doctor not doing his job, my husband started saying the same thing the doctor did for that two and a half year period of time. I cannot tell you the torture of something like that. To trust someone you love, and have them turn their back on you, call you "sick in the head" for years, steals a person's positive energy necessary to fight these health battles. It's exhausting to try to tell someone who is supposed to love you, and know you, that things are not in your head. It's exhausting, having to tell the people who are supposed to have your back, that you feel as bad as you do, and need their support.

The things I have lived through, I would not wish on my worst enemy. Living with, and around someone who is inflicted with this disease requires patience, understanding, compassion, and most of all, love. Support is imperative. Going to the doctor alone is a "no-no." Bit by bit, my family's refusal to believe me, and the inability to function properly, grew to a devastating level. The close bond I shared with my daughter was crushed.

No one wanted to go to the doctor with me for years during the time everyone was telling me my health was in my head. Trying to get anyone to give me the support I needed, as opposed to what everyone decided I needed, was a battle that always left me feeling sicker and worn out. Everyone was too busy with their schedules to work together on a regular basis to help with the doctors and hospitals. I constantly asked for help to call doctors, to help find a doctor who knew about Gastroparesis. I needed someone to help me with scheduling, keeping things organized, and getting to doctors. I heard excuses like, "I can't do any more than you are doing." "I don't have time for this." "I don't want to hear about your illness." "It's not always about you," etc., etc. I just wish they would have been able to see the health problems even though I didn't look as sick on the outside.

Inside, we are still the same people. These illnesses are painful, can be life threatening, and can become fatal at any point, if severe. Support from those who are supposed to be our families, our loved ones, our safety net, is imperative when you are this sick. From where I stand, I don't see much in the way of family support or a safety net. I'm not saying that people in my family do not do things. I am saying, it is scattered, never consistent, and never a plan of action or enough support to actually get me to the point of functioning in a safe, clean home, with doctors who know what is going on with these different illnesses. A plant of action, so I can function to the best of my ability, on a daily basis, and have some sense of independence.

Something I could never understand, was how Mike respected the doctor's opinion, as opposed to the everyday visual appearance of how sick I was getting and how much help I needed just to function. When I would try to talk to Mike and tell him how sick I was, he would say, "Yeah, sick in the head." When I would cry he turned his back on me, which was daily, and told me I needed to be committed to a psych ward. He would then walk away leaving me frustrated and hanging on the edge. Being chronically ill is not a walk in the park for either spouse. It is difficult to watch your spouse decline and fight to live.

This is a horrible illness to live with and when those around you add negative stress to your life instead of support and smiles, it makes you feel so much worse. Family is supposed to love one another and support one another through everything. Good and bad. It is not all good, but to love those who are in your life through everything, shows your own honest commitment to love. It is so important to keep talking with each other through difficult times. Don't expect the problems to go away on their own. Problems become elephants in the room if they aren't discussed. Everyone knows about the problem, but all too often, responsibility is not taken to correct it and the problem continues.

Those who depend on God for support and guidance seem to have a different attitude and strength. *Faith* and *hope* are two very important qualities a person can possess. Through *hope* comes determination, and through *faith* comes the strength to keep going. To all families who are going through medical difficulties, put your trust in God. Believe what your family members who are sick are saying to you about how they are feeling. Try to find a way to better understand, so the difficulties of these illnesses can be easier lived and fought together. Have *faith* that the truth is being told by the family member who is sick and have *hope* that you can change the situation.

119

Hope and *faith* will also bring the determination needed to fight the tough battles. Doctors are people who went to school deciding on a medical field of employment. They are sworn to always help others and "first do no harm." Those of us going through chronic illnesses know that an oath may be sworn to, but that does not mean that an oath is always kept. By not listening, harm can be done.

I don't know that my family has a way back from the direction it is headed, but I remain *hope*ful. I'm the only one who seems to want everyone to sit down together, in the same room, and actually talk. Begin working on forgiving one another as opposed to constant negative actions and attitudes. Don't expect to be forgiven for walking over people constantly, if you pretend you do nothing and never ask to be forgiven. People get tired of being walked on, even if it is the family they love. Each one of us in any situation experiences life in his, or her, own way. We can be there to support one another, and that is so important, but as similar as so many situations seem to be, there are just as many differences. No two people, no two lives, are ever the same.

It is so important to respect the differences of each other, whether we are sick or not. Our differences make up our uniqueness, our individuality. We are all special and each person has their own strengths. Through working together, respecting one another, we can use those differences along with the similarities to create balance and peace. I've met many people who feel they have the most to offer and those who don't think they are good enough to offer anything. Both types of people are equally as important and have different perspectives. I believe through working together, having the ability to understand one another, by bringing the similarities and differences together, can create relationships that can stand united and perhaps understand situations on a broader level.

Communication is the key in any type of relationship, or group. Can you imagine a support group without communication? Or a mother and daughter buying school supplies, unable to communicate with each other. They would need the support of a third party to relay information in order to purchase anything at all. Unless we have the ability to communicate in any situation, family, friend, patient/physician relationship, the relationship will always fail. Communication in any relationship is like water to plants, without it, they cannot survive.

During the First Annual Health Care Summit held in DC in 2012, I had most of my research confirmed, but found out many other important pieces of information. There is only a 55% success ratio with the patient/physician relationship. I would imagine communication has quite a bit to do with that, and I don't mean on the patient's part. So many doctors do not want to listen or hear what their patients are saying to them about what they are feeling. They sit there, looking at you in judgment, as opposed to realizing there are many things going on in the world that doctors do not understand or even know about. Most doctors do things according to protocol, or better known as "working in a box." This eliminates so much of the population. Many of us who are sick do not fit in these boxes.

Those in the medical community, first and foremost, need to learn how to listen and communicate. To take an oath to help others, and then pick and choose who gets the help, isn't that judging and playing God? A doctor is supposed to care about the well-being of others. Not pick and choose who gets the care. Not label people who question or challenge what is being said, with names like depression, anxiety, social anxiety disorder, eating disorder, drug seeker, hypochondriac, that ends up on your record for all in the medical field to see. Doctors are allowed to label us if they are having a bad day or do not like what we are saying, and there is nothing we can do about it. I have tried. I have been through it, along with so many others that I have come to know. I had no idea how much this kind of thing went on, until I had to face it myself. I even hired a psychiatrist and a counselor who handles drug dependency as well. Hiring them was the best thing I could have ever done for myself. There are many people in this field as well. When choosing any type of doctor, remember that they are people. People who can either help or hurt you. Your life is important. We are all important. People should be able to stand up for themselves and speak out, without being judged.

My daughter was a straight "A" student, until I became too sick to function. From the time Sam was born, she had a mother she could depend on, who was strong and stood up for what was right, not what was easy. She had a mom she could depend on to be there, even when she didn't want her to be. I made plenty of mistakes, but I was a good mom. Then, within the blink of an eye, she had a mom who she couldn't depend on any longer. I do not know how she feels inside, but I am sure that it must have been torture to have to endure all of the things I had to go through, as well as what she had to go through, without the proper support. She didn't want to see me hurt any more than I wanted to hurt. During an emergency visit she had to go with me to the hospital, she cried because I screamed from the pain of the nurse slicing my leg and twisting to squeeze out infection that was not there to squeeze out. I had a staph infection that started to take my leg out and cutting it open made it worse. I have experienced entirely too many types of pain in this life.

With Dr. X telling me so much of what was happening was in my head, my daughter was infuriated. She was growing up without the family support all children should have. I do know that at the age of sixteen, Sam planned my granddaughter and married her first love. I do know that neither

Samantha, nor her husband were ready to be parents, but inside she had to have been terrified to be left in this world alone if I died. She felt like I already left her at that point. I do know that the beautiful incredible smile she used to have, disappeared completely. I do know that she has cried endless amounts of tears and I can only assume she doesn't want to feel the fear and pain of me being this sick, so she stays angry instead. I miss snuggling up and watching a movie with her. What Sam doesn't understand is that she makes my heart peaceful and happy. When she is peaceful and happy, I am peaceful and happy. She is my baby and always will be. She and my granddaughter are the twinkle in my eye and the extra push in my step. Sam and Carissa are pieces of my heart and soul that make me who I am. Because of being sick, I could no longer be the mother I was and wanted to continue to be. I can never be the grandma I want to be. I am a wonderful grandma, for what I am able to do! I love being a grandma, but I could be so much more if I was not fighting so much pain, nausea, weakness and other debilitating things that go along with this body. To push your body when it says it just cannot go anymore truly makes you appreciate every second that you have of your life.

The disconnect with my family grew more and more as I worked from my hospital bed on designing and developing the organization, Teen Moms Fresh Start. My daughter was a teen mom by the time my colon was removed. I wasn't sure what was going to happen to me. I already had to fight for my life, and the doctors had no idea what to do. In the hospital and out, I researched programs for her to attend. I was horrified at what was happening in our country. If I died, I was afraid there would be nothing for Sam and Carissa that would offer everything a person would need to become independent and confident. In 2008, I created Teen Moms Friends Club, Inc., (also doing business as, dba) Teen Moms Fresh Start, which is a 501c3 Nonprofit based in Maryland. I thought if other people could be there during situations that I would not be able to be, she would be safer than trying to figure out how life worked alone. I worked from my bed at home. I went to meetings when I felt up to it. We had begun workshops, helping those in need of food, clothing, furniture items, Christmas and Thanksgiving needs, as well as birthdays.

While I may have been very sick during this time period, it was important to me to help as much as possible. After I found out all of the different types of issues that were happening in the teen world, seeing the lack of education and support that was so needed to change what was happening, I had to keep going. Helping others helped me stay alive. Fighting for your life with a chronic illness is probably one of the most difficult tasks that can be thrown into a person's life. As long as I kept looking forward, kept talking to God and letting him guide me, I knew I could keep going. I knew I could and I did. Through Teen Moms Fresh Start, we helped many families until I had come to a standstill. Too many hospitalizations, fevers, blood infections, and then some. Even in the hospital, after we temporarily stopped workshops, I still made sure to help a couple of families with Christmas and Thanksgiving.

During all of this time, I tried to include Sam so that she would have the benefit of the workshops, meeting other teen moms, as well as something we could do together that was positive, as opposed to negative sick times. The sicker I became, the more she backed away. At one point, when I was 94 pounds, she looked at me for a second and then said she couldn't stand to look at me and ran out of the house. She left shortly after to go to a friend's house. The entire last six years has been exceptionally difficult on all of us. I think my daughter especially because we used to be so close, and I protected her from everything I could until I couldn't protect her anymore.

My family saw me work on Teen Moms Fresh Start, and judged me deciding that I wasn't sick enough if I was working on Teen Moms. Not one person in my family would listen to the fact that doing the right thing was keeping me alive. Sam needed just as much support as everyone else who was in her shoes, and I wished she would have joined in with the groups and activities. She was so angry at me for developing and working on the organization, as opposed to putting all of my focus on taking care of her and Carissa the way she thought I should, our relationship was wearing down even further. Sam began to resent what I was doing.

From the very beginning, my husband wasn't happy about the organization either, which encouraged Samantha to be negative. In my opinion, embarrassment was more of an issue than anything for Mike. He wasn't embarrassed to be with Sam or Carissa, he was embarrassed over the words "teen moms." He seemed to have the attitude resembling many people I have met during events, festivals, meetings, etc, who shrug or blow off, who act rude and offensive when it comes to the topic of teen pregnancy. Mike did not believe in me, which added obstacles. He has not seen all of the things that I have done, all of the things that I had to do in order to eat, live, teach and raise my daughter when I was a single parent. I was a single mom for 14 years.

When the colon was removed March 20, 2008, our family began a rapid decent, like a plane nose diving. I actually lost *hope* for a very brief moment. I had been through too much in my life at that point. I had no idea I could actually lose *hope*, but one night I did. During that brief moment, that one night, I thought this was it. There was no way out of the ruins and devastation created from being this sick. I was being accused of faking all of the symptoms I was having, by my own family. The medical professionals I was seeing were telling me it was in my head even after the removal of my colon. I had become weak, in bed constantly, throwing up, uncontrollable diarrhea, I could not take it anymore. My uncle had passed away. My grandparents had passed. Sam was going through so much she turned her back on me. Mike did not believe me, and put me down constantly. I had lost *hope*, but only for a moment. I now know what so many others feel like who have lost *hope*. During much of my life, as difficult as it had been, I had not lost *hope*. Never in my life, at any point, did I think that I would not have tomorrow to get to my feet and fight for what is right. As hard as things were, I would keep fighting, putting one foot in front of the other, never giving up.

I raised Sam by myself, from the time she was a year old. I had to overcome quite a bit as a single parent, but during all of that time, I never lost *hope*. While I fought being sick every day prior to being hospitalized and housebound, I had not been that sick before. I never had to depend on anyone the way I had to depend on my family at this point. I did so much for my family prior to becoming sick, but now I could no longer function properly. Many times, the things that I did to help were forgotten, as if I had been this disabled my entire life. Doing things in return wasn't their strong suit, but then I did not do for them to get anything in return. I did it because I wanted to. Perhaps they didn't want me to be sick, so maybe they didn't want to believe it. Or perhaps they didn't want to handle responsibilities so denying I was that sick was the easiest way for them to handle life. I'm not them, I don't know what they were feeling. Only they do and God. They refused to talk anymore. No one planned anything. Everyone ran in different directions and I was the one stuck holding the bag every day, alone at home, when I needed help.

Life seems to be getting more difficult on a daily basis. I lose more strength and endurance, as well as become sicker for a period. I end up having to get used to it if I want to live and function. Each step taken with these illnesses has been very difficult, but you learn to live with what you have and continue to go on another day. I thank God for every day, including that one night I lost *hope*. I know He was there to carry me through and teach me something beautiful. God does not let us go down paths we cannot recover from when we walk in *faith*. That doesn't mean you ask for something and if you don't get it then God isn't listening. That is not *faith* at all. That is the furthest example of *faith* because there is no belief, or *faith*, to begin with. It's as if those type of people don't believe they are going to get what they ask for anyway, so they chalk it up to no one listening and go on living the same way.

Some people only ask God for help when circumstances seem so bleak that death or disaster is imminent. Circumstances that may seem unbearable for a time, for me anyway, have always ended up showing me something I may have never seen otherwise. I am able to understand how horrible it is to be bound by something that you cannot physically overcome, and be subdued by everyone and everything around you. I was able to come back from that and tell everyone that it is so important never to lose *hope* or *faith*. Those are two very important attributes that keep our spirit strong and alive. If we don't keep our eyes on God, we can lose our way very easily. Staying focused on doing the right thing, believing that things are okay no matter what circumstances tell us, asking God for the strength to go on and give back along the way, is all a part of keeping our eyes on God. I know the only way I have made it through some very difficult times is to keep my eyes forward. Always keeping my eyes on God, asking Him and thanking Him for the strength and courage He gives to me.

My relationship with my husband changed completely. Mike stopped looking at me the same. I became a burden as opposed to someone of strength he could depend on as well. Someone who would be there for him so he would not be alone. Someone he could spend life with having fun. When someone is halted in their tracks by something that stops their body from functioning, the part of "In Sickness and In Health" vows should be kicking in. Helping to find a way to make life livable while dealing with the health issues.

I hear of too many who leave their spouses due to illness. It is awful when someone blames you for being sick. It is exhausting to be sick. But to be sick and beg your spouse to believe you, is almost like not having a light at the end of the tunnel. The trust is demolished. The emptiness can be overwhelming. *Faith*, and my relationship with

God, has been the only thing that has kept me going. I know when we call God, he hears us. We may not always receive the outcome we want, but in the larger scheme of things, when I look back at my own life's trials and tribulations, everything came in its time and in perfect order. I do not blame anyone for why I am sick, especially God. I know that He has helped me stay here to do whatever I can to let others know what is happening with all of these health issues. It is difficult to do when you are so weak, but when I ask God to fill me with His strength to do what I need to do, He helps me get things done.

I used to push myself too far doing research to find a way to get better. I post the research so others can see on GastroparesisAndME.com, GPnMEGlobal.org, and other social networking sites. By doing that, education is available for those who do not know where to go to begin. I know there is so much more information out there that still needs to be found and posted so these illnesses are given the attention they should have so those who are dealing with this can get the care and respect so overdue and deserved. This also allows anyone to build on that research, hopefully bringing us closer every day to answers and a cure. I do get knocked off my feet multiple times a week. Those are the times I sleep the deepest. Because of the chronic symptoms, I do not ever get to sleep through the night. Neither does Mike.

###

Colossians 3:18-21

Wives, be subject to your husbands [out of respect for their position as protector, and their accountability to God], as is proper and fitting in the Lord. Husbands, love your wives [with an affectionate, sympathetic, selfless love that always seeks the best for them] and do not be embittered or resentful toward them [because of the responsibilities of marriage]. Children, obey your parents [as God's representatives] in all things, for this [attitude of respect and obedience] is well-pleasing to the Lord [and will bring you God's promised blessings]. Fathers, do not provoke or irritate or exasperate your children [with demands that are trivial or unreasonable or humiliating or abusive; nor by favoritism or indifference; treat them tenderly with loving kindness], so they will not lose heart and become discouraged or unmotivated [with their sprits broken].

Chapter 7

What? Look, I've Got Muscles!

I didn't know anyone else who had GP, so at first I thought it must be rare. I had never heard of it in my many visits with multiple doctors or the over abundant hospital stays. I knew I needed to learn as much about this as I could. I certainly didn't know that I would end up meeting some of the most incredible people, in this country and out, who are very sick as well. I had no idea that I would find that there are millions of people fighting for their lives. I had no idea that I would make some incredible friends, and then lose them to these illnesses. When I first started looking into this, I had no idea that I was about to find out how much devastation this brings to so many others.

A big test of my *faith* and strength came in December when a terrible flu hit me. It hit so hard, that I honestly wasn't sure that I was going to make it through. Mike had already gone to work when the fever hit. That left me home alone with Carissa, who was three at the time. On a good day, I needed a walker or a wheelchair during this time period. My legs had become weak from losing muscle mass and from fighting multiple blood infections. But on this day, I could not get out of bed. I felt so horrible, that even touching the ends of my hair hurt from the fever. I had to call Mike and have him come home. It took him a bit, but I was so thankful when he did get home. I was able to rest, instead of trying to talk to Carissa to keep her occupied so she wouldn't get into things she shouldn't.

My fever would not break with Tylenol and ice the first two days. The first day was the roughest. While Mike was downstairs, I had no way of calling out to him. I had gotten too weak. I was in and out of deep sleep. After a while, I started feeling like I couldn't open my eyes or move my body anymore. I couldn't call out to Mike, my body wouldn't let me.

Mike had pulled away from me several of years before the flu hit, so he stopped checking on me and caring the way he had. I was laying there, all alone. Just God and I. I felt like I just wanted to go home at that point. I was too sick to be left alone for hours at a time. No one seemed to care. My daughter separated herself, my husband separated himself, my grandparents had passed. My grandparents love me unconditionally, and did so much for me, and with me, while they were alive.

I was having problems breathing, it was becoming too exhausting and my body felt like it just didn't have the energy to keep going. I asked God to please bring me home; to please separate me from this body that had become a torture chamber. I wanted to go home and be at peace. I have been sick a very long time. Peace is something that gets disrupted with the jolts of pain, nausea, vomiting, and other debilitating symptoms. I just didn't want to keep suffering anymore. Ultimately, I knew it was not my time. There was still too much to do here and it was not time for me to go yet.

Thank God for all of the natural plants and herbs He has given us to help ourselves with. Thank God for giving us the knowledge to understand the benefits of nature, as well as the natural energy of the earth. While we are busy running to doctors to find answers as to why something is happening to us, there are many proactive things we can do to help ourselves stay as healthy as we can. When we are young, we exercise to get in shape, look good, and of course, feel good. But when all of your energy becomes stripped away from health problems, or even age, you begin to look in other directions when conventional medicine does not work.

I have always been a healthy eater, of course snacking on sweet things sometimes, but for the most part a healthy eater. I had to watch what I ate because so much of what contained preservatives in processed foods made me sick. My stomach wasn't very cooperative as far back as I can remember. It gradually worsened as time went on.

During one of my hospital stays, I had to work from my phone to set up a table at an event at Timonium Fairgrounds in Maryland. The event was the "World of Possibilities Expo." A friend of mine, Mona Freedman, who is the founder of *Caring Communities*, created the World of Possibilities Expo, and many other incredible community events to help others. I was very disappointed when I was unable to attend the Expo that year due to my health. While I may have missed a very important meeting that day, the person I was supposed to meet contacted me and came to visit me at the Greater Baltimore Medical Center where I was hospitalized. She also ended up becoming my friend, Pam Gecan. Thanks Pam.

Pam brought some energy wellness products with her to the hospital. I had been on and off of IV nutrition for several years at that point, and was having so many complications. I didn't realize Pam's main interests revolved around our bodies and natural healthy support, as opposed to conventional medicine to be healthier. That was right up my alley. I was interested in exactly the same thing, but everything I had used up to that point did not reduce the nausea the way I needed. It did not help keep me out of the hospital. It did not help maintain strength nor provide me with what I needed to function. I wanted to get better, but traditional medicine was not helping. In most cases, medicines made things worse. If you are a Poor Metabolizer of most medications, it is near impossible to find a medication that does not cause allergic reactions to severe adverse reactions. In fact, many of them can cause death if it is a medication you cannot metabolize. Poor Metabolism is a genetic issue.

During that stay, May of 2011, a few things happened. First, the products that Pam had brought settled my stomach more than any medication I had ever been given for nausea. More than any other homeopathic remedies I have tried. I was thankful to have my nausea reduced some. The chronic nausea is like having food poisoning or a bad flu that never ends. I was amazed that something actually helped.

Second, the gastroenterologist sat in my room, after I was told that I was going to have genetic testing to see what was going on, and then preceded to tell me that I would do better in a different medical facility. The genetic testing was not going to take place and I would need to find other doctors. I could not believe what I was hearing. Pam and my mother were there that day. I felt like I was the punch line of some type of horrible torturous joke. I went from thinking this geneticist could help me find some answers, to what in the world was I going to do now. I had to find another group of doctors, explain everything all over again, which becomes tiresome after a while, and hope someone would listen. I was doing everything healthy that I could think of while trying to find answers in the medical profession.

Toward the end of 2011, I had decided that I was going to sign a DNR (Do Not Resuscitate) and never go on IV nutrition again. I was so tired of being sick. I was so tired of people telling me everything was in my head or that I was a drug seeker. I was worn out from trying to convince almost every doctor I scheduled with that I was sick and needed help finding out what was going on, before I lost all of my energy or my life. I couldn't go through these horrible hospitalizations. And for what? To be called a drug seeker??

Having a history of IV nutrition, colonic inertia, my colon removed, Ulcerative Colitis, vomiting that required Botox injections inside of the stomach at the pyloric area, I thought that was enough information to find a new doctor to replace Dr. X. Almost no one wanted to help. I had to hear the typical comments, "Too complicated," "What do you want me to do?" and "I don't specialize in that. You will have to find someone who specializes in that area." It makes me wonder if doctors are really into being doctors more for the money, rather than helping people with serious illnesses get better. There may be many expenses associated with being a doctor, however, there are many more expenses for those who are chronically ill.

If a doctor is allowed to say, "I don't know enough about that," and continue to be part of the problem by staying uneducated, as opposed to part of the solution, where will this end? Too many lives have been lost due to lack of education, and too many more are fighting in many ways to live. It is important physicians listen to their patients.

We know our bodies and what is happening inside of us.

It is important that doctors work together, with the patient, when it comes to a patient's needs, as well as work with one another for the best outcome possible. It is equally as important to work with other doctors who are working with the patients. Whether they are familiar with a particular physician or not, by working together, the patient's with medical care will be greatly improved. Many patients make comments that their doctors aren't listening to what they are saying. Instead of these ridiculous psychological labels, or drug seeking labels that are placed in a person's medical records causing all kinds of problems with new doctors or hospital visits, listen to patients and help them make it through this.

A huge number of people living with these illnesses ask for pain medication because it is unbearable pain that knocks you on the floor or keeps you in bed in a ball. Try to find the source of the pain, weakness, and other oddities, as opposed to labeling. That is no different than stereotyping and acting in a prejudiced and discriminatory manner. We talk about racial, ethnic, and other discrimination and prejudices. We don't talk about the discrimination medical patients face when dealing with the medical professionals. We want the discrimination and stereotyping to end and the truth to take its place so we can receive the help we need.

After surviving the flu, I knew if I was going to continue to live and be able to research to understand and help break the silence that hovers over these illnesses, I was going to need to get my body stronger. On January 6, 2012, I began using energy wellness products. God did not create everything on this earth just to look at; there are many types of plants and herbs we can use to help ourselves. Several companies have found ways to use exactly what God gave us to benefit ourselves. The company that Pam introduced me to was

ZeroPoint Global. I was in a wheelchair or using a walker toward the end of 2011, depending upon how I felt that day. I had lost the muscles in my legs that resulted in two separate eight week stretches of physical therapy, which did not help at all.

Nothing before that time seemed to be helping. I tried so hard, but my muscles didn't want to keep going. After the first four days of using multiple products from ZeroPoint Global, I was off of the walker and out of the wheelchair! I did not change anything in my regular daily routine. After six weeks of using the ZeroPoint Global products, I had muscles in my legs and even did a deep knee bend! Mike was the first to notice I had muscles in my legs. He looked at my legs and said, "Look, you have muscles!" I looked and realized I did have muscles again. I did not do anything different. Nothing, other than use the energy wellness products. What an incredible triumph that was. An amazing incredible feeling to be able to walk again and actually do a deep knee bend.

This was such an encouraging event. During my physical therapy sessions, we had to put pillows on the chair that gave me about 2 inches of room to stand up and sit down. I used to just drop down onto the chair, so it was impossible to do exercises without the pillows. I went from not being able to walk up and down the steps without help, to walking very quickly up and down the stairs if I needed to. It was complete freedom. These are my personal experiences that I am sharing, and I am in no way offering any type of medical advice, or saying this will do the same for everyone.

While I was able to get around, I was still in pain, nauseous, and still having some weak spells, but I was able to get around again. I wanted to go dancing, go out and have fun. There were many things I wanted to do that I didn't quite have the energy for. I was beginning to have the energy to function quite a bit better. As long as I used the Mint Matrix, the nausea went down. I used the lasers on my food and on me. I wore the Sirius Balance Pendant. I used the ClearingSET to help clear any trauma to the body, conscious or unconscious. I used the smaller frequency discs on locations that were in pain, and actually experienced pain relief in some areas. I used the larger frequency discs to sit food on and energize. I currently put all of my IV nutrition bags on one of the large frequency discs to energize what I am bringing in to help my body. I used the Sirius Silver which helped reduce the number of colds and flus I picked up. My family also used it, which kept us all feeling better, making life a bit easier.

The ZeroPoint Global products are a blessing. One day my granddaughter had gotten poison ivy. I washed her hands and put the Citrus Silk on it before she went to bed. I also put the clay that is infused with sound frequencies and energy frequencies, along with the Sirius Silver to make a paste. I used the red natural laser for about 2 minutes. I put the band aid on and off to sleep she went. In the morning when we got up, she took off the band aid and the poison ivy that takes several weeks to heal, was already beginning to dry up. I was wowed. Carissa was so happy that she was not itching. Ever since that day, Carissa will reach for whichever product, depending on what she needs them for. The red natural laser coagulated the blood when she sliced her pinky finger. You could see the blood stop and a deep dark line form on her finger where the cut was. She sliced it good and ever since then, if anyone gets a cut, the red natural laser comes out, the Sirius Silver, and then the band aids. They are truly remarkable products and so easy to use that my 6 year old granddaughter knows what to grab for a boo boo or poison ivy.

There are so many uses for each one of the energy products. This is an area traditional doctors don't seem to like to discuss, and many don't seem to believe in. None that I have spoken with yet anyway. I don't understand how this is possible, since doctors are always telling you to eat healthy and exercise to stay fit. Energy wellness support is just like eating healthy and exercising. The natural way to a stronger you. If I didn't experience it for myself, I'm not sure if I would have believed it. I'm fortunate Pam showed me the different energy wellness products, along with so many other healthy conversations we have had. Anytime I found anything through my research that was worth discussing, I would bring it up. Vice versa. If Pam found anything that was helpful, she would let me know.

It is important to talk to as many people as possible when it comes to our health. Please advocate for yourself and know that we are all human. Including doctors. We all make mistakes, including doctors. I know I have my share of forgiving to do. If any of the doctors who turned me away, telling me I looked good, would have listened and helped me through this, I know I wouldn't be so short fused when it comes to those who work in the medical profession. It is important that we continue to educate and share information whenever and however possible because I've lost too many friends due to these illnesses. I am so tired of hearing that someone else passed away, and I am tired of fighting every day to live.

###

Proverbs 3:5-8

Trust in and rely confidently on the Lord with all your heart and do not rely on your own insight or understanding. In all your ways know and acknowledge and recognize Him, and He will make your paths straight and smooth [removing obstacles that block your way]. Do not be wise in your own eyes; Fear the Lord [with reverent awe and obedience] and turn [entirely] away from evil. It will be health to your body [your marrow, your nerves, your sinews, your muscles – all your inner parts] and refreshment (physical well-being) to your bones.

Chapter 8

Is There a Doctor in the Country?

When I began writing this book, prior to being diagnosed, I was wondering if there was a doctor in the country who could figure out what was wrong with me. Hence the name, "Is There a Doctor in the Country?" All of the doctors I had seen told me everything was in my head. I knew things weren't in my head, they were in my guts, skeletal system, muscles and the rest of my body. I didn't think there was anyone in the country who knew about all of the symptoms I was experiencing and having to live with.

Imagine decades of doctor visits, only to hear the same thing over and over, "You are depressed, you have anxiety, you have an eating disorder," or some other statement that opposes what you know; that there is something physically wrong and it's not getting better. You cannot help but develop anger toward those who are pointing fingers instead of helping. It's not worth it to be angry, but I was. I was very angry by all the years that have gone by. Doctors looking at the word *depression* and blowing me off. When one doctor puts something in your record, getting it out is unbearable. Not impossible, just unbearable having to go through everything you have to in order to get your medical records fixed.

By the time I was in my 30s, I was furious with the medical profession in general. Every time I went to a new doctor, explaining how I was feeling, I would always get the "but you look so good" comment. I didn't care how good I looked, I felt like I was dying. I felt like my body was being destroyed and I was worn out constantly. Even though I was worn out, I was still able to take care of my daughter, my granddaughter, and the household responsibilities early on when my granddaughter was born. Prior to that, when my daughter was growing up, I was able to be a single parent, even though I didn't have the strength that so many other people had. I pushed extra hard with everything. If I wanted a life, I had to work for it every day. I am so grateful for who I am and for knowing how important it is to trust in God and to trust ourselves no matter what anyone says.

When you know something isn't right, don't let a doctor tell you otherwise. Who knows your body better than yourself? There are too many people who have been misdiagnosed with one thing or another. People are people no matter what position they hold, so it is an injustice to yourself not to trust yourself. You are your best advocate. It is also so important to make sure when you go to a doctor appointment that you take someone with you every time. Being alone in any situation is not good. If problems should occur, the situation becomes your word against someone else's word. If you have someone with you, you have a witness. More often than not, should a doctor have a problem with you personally or the medical problems you are experiencing, as long as you have someone with you, the condescending words, nasty angry attitudes, patronizing tones and words remain restrained.

Last year, I saw a doctor at Hopkins in Baltimore. He was my personal physician for a short time. It was during a time that I needed to be back on IV nutrition, but no one would listen. I had dropped to 94 pounds. My heart was pounding through my breast bone like someone beating down a door. My heart beat consumed my entire body and I knew if I didn't get nutrition soon, I was not going to be able to survive the starvation. This doctor used the name of Hopkins as his reference for the reason he could be so judgmental and why I was the moron patient who knew nothing. My lungs were exhausted and worse than usual. My oxygen was 87 percent, so I took some of the shallow quick breaths I have learned to do to keep my oxygen higher when I cannot breathe. It went up to 94/95 percent, so they documented that for the O2 saturation levels as opposed to the original 87 percent. They did this because they knew the doctor was going to let me go that evening. I was so sick, I actually thought I was going in that day to talk about getting back on the IV nutrition, until I arrived to find all of the attitudes around me. At that point I knew what they were doing, so I had to at least attempt to get this doctor to listen to how important it was for me to get back on the TPN so that I could get the hydration, nutrition, and weight I needed.

Pam was actually with me on that occasion. She knew there was nothing that was going to change this doctor's mind. So she sat and listened while I talked to him to try to get him to see how much I needed this. There was no breaking through the "I'm right, you are wrong, and I don't feel like dealing with you" attitude. Here I am, fighting for my life, and this man just throws me away like a piece of trash, and used the institution he works for as his backbone of strength. I have found that to be the case concerning many doctors at Hopkins.

I am only just beginning to meet doctors affiliated with Hopkins who actually believe they are human and not above me because of their position. I have found this to be a pleasant and much needed change. Too many times, when reputations grow too large, many are lost in the cracks because of the lack of accountability. After experiencing what I have in my life, as well as finding out I am not the only one this is happening to, all over our country, at an alarming rate. I feel it is important that more and more people continue to speak out. Hopefully this will eventually begin to change. It has been because of the lack of knowledge that many people living with these type of Silent Illnesses have lost their lives. Friends and family are left devastated wondering why their loved one had to die; wondering why more people in the medical industry do not know about Gastroparesis, Ehlers-Danlos,

Dysautonomia, Chiari Malformation, and so on. Why is there such a struggle to get medical professionals to believe what a patient is telling them. Why does this have to be so difficult?

Dr. X, who I spent entirely too many years trying to convince I was sick and not depressed, decided a couple of years ago that I was not getting the help I needed through him and it was time to find a new doctor. I agreed with him as well. Unfortunately, leaving Dr. X prior to finding a doctor who was educated in the areas I needed sent me bouncing from doctor to doctor. When that happened, I began being accused of doctor jumping which gave doctors another excuse for them not to help. This has not stopped. I have not found another personal physician yet, and hope I am sure I am on my way to finding the right person. Ever since being labelled a Demerol seeker, I have yet to find a doctor who listens to me as opposed to the red flags that are now in my medical records. One of the doctors I was referred to by Dr. X, who was to look for Crohn's or some other explanation for the digestive problems I was having, wrote in his notes that I was continuing Demerol seeking behavior. How in the world, in one visit, never seeing this doctor before, could he have ever thought I was a Demerol seeker if my doctor hadn't said something to that effect? This physician, as all others in the medical profession who take medical history, asked me if I had any allergies. My answer, as it always has been, is most antibiotics I have previously been given, sulfa drugs, and a number of other drugs in the narcotic family, with the exception of Demerol. All of these medications cause my body to react negatively, and I refuse to take them. In no way does that indicate I am continuing to exhibit Demerol seeking behavior.

I was in an emergency room one time for whatever was happening with the Gastroparesis, when I asked the ER doctor to call Dr. X about the Demerol. I asked him to talk to Dr. X because he knew I couldn't take anything but that without a reaction. Well, that's what I thought at the time. The doctor in the emergency room came back to say that Dr. X was leaving the medication up to the emergency room doctor. I was so upset and in so much pain. Dr. X had the nerve to call me a whiny woman with depression on multiple occasions, as well as left me laying on his office floor in agony, after a horrible jolt of pain from my gall bladder knocked me right off the patient table. Gall bladder pain can be unbearable. So there I was, living with all of this pain, trying to get basic healthcare to find out what was wrong, so that I could function, but no one would listen or help.

There have been many other negative situations with Dr. X, yet he was still paid for each and every visit. He was paid for his time, but I did not get proper medical care in return for the money I had to pay him. No sympathy, help or compassion from this doctor, and I was no better off for the money and visits I spent with him. Instead, I now have a history of being a drug-seeking, doctor hopping, whiny, depressed individual – shit out of luck!! Living with GP isn't easy!!

Dr. X tried to convince Mike to commit me to an institution during one visit a number of years ago. He told Mike all of this was in my head, which also caused incredible problems in our marriage. Dr. X said and did many other neglectful, emotionally abusive things prior to me leaving, that I dealt with. He was also the doctor who prescribed the Demerol for me while I was his patient, through surgeries and procedures. Almost all of the doctors he sent me to also said nothing was wrong. It was a very frustrating nine years. The cardiologist he sent me to within his practice, was actually screaming in my face that there was nothing wrong with my heart. When I told Dr. X about the situation, he laughed and said that sounds like him sometimes. That was all he said or did about that.

After I left Dr. X, I saw another cardiologist who was not affiliated with his practice in any way. My current cardiologist, over the past five or six years, found that I have tachycardia due to Dysautonomia. This was one of the reasons I was feeling so horrible. I stayed with that cardiologist for several years, who followed me and made sure I was okay. As I mentioned previously, I started seeing Dr. Clair Francomano, who is the geneticist at Greater Baltimore Medical Center. From the very first visit with Dr. Francomano, she listened to me. I have never felt like a doctor ever truly listened or tried to understand anything I ever said I was experiencing. For years, doctors told me I was depressed. That was the easy way out for too many years. The gastroenterologists Dr. X sent me to see found nothing but mild gastritis. One of the doctors he sent me to in 2005, did find that my stomach was emptying entirely too slow, but nothing was done. A delay of 262 minutes in emptying my stomach into my intestines. Prior to faxing him, I even wrote on the document about the delayed gastric emptying possibly being a culprit of what was happening, and perhaps lead us to what was going on with me. Not once was that document addressed. I did not receive proper medical care the entire time I was with Dr. X, as I have come to find out. After leaving him, the gall bladder that needed to come out for quite some time was finally removed. That was an incredible relief that stopped me from dropping to the floor from jabs of pain.

I had no idea the majority of the reason I was not receiving proper care was because this doctor had decided I was a fake, and he was not going to treat me according to what I was telling him. That was so wrong, and unless physicians are held accountable for everything they do, what I and many others have lived through will continue. Doctors are human too.

Temple University found out in January of 2008 that I had Gastroparesis and Colonic Inertia. I wasn't aware of this finding until 2011. When I look back on everything that has transpired throughout my entire life, I am definitely a part of the 45% of the patient/physician relationships that are not getting the help needed to function and live. The panelists introduced that number during the First Annual Health Care Summit held at The Chamber of Commerce in DC, 2012. In 2013, I was too sick to make it to the second Summit. I wanted to be there to hear what was going on so that I could make notes to add to the research I am doing. It is extremely important that physicians are held accountable for everything they do, regardless of the excuses that are given. Too many patients end up being treated subhuman, like I had been treated on countless occasions.

One time during an emergency room visit, someone I know who is in the public eye came to see me. When he came into my room, I let him know how bad they were treating me. He told me I didn't look so great and I told him I would get through, as I always do. His presence in my room changed everything. The doctors and nurses treated me as if I was the President of the United States or the Queen of England. It made me sick to see how these people changed because of the popularity of someone else. I was given more attention, in addition to higher quality attention, just because he was there and has had his picture taken in many places, with many people, doing community activities, volunteer work, etc. Things I wish I could still be doing as well. My entire life I have been helping others. I have taken care of family members, sacrificed everything I wanted and needed to raise my daughter, on my own. I took care of my grandmom before she died. I've tried to do right by people, whether I know them or not. Those people taking care of me in the emergency room only cared that this person I knew was popular. They weren't concerned for my welfare. If I had not experienced it myself, I would not have known what it feels like to actually receive good to excellent treatment in a hospital or doctor setting. My friend laughed, but I did not find this funny at all. I found it to be horribly poor behavior that certain people receive better treatment than others simply because of who they are. My life is equally as important! If medical professionals are able to treat me better because of someone in the public eye, then they are able to treat me right because I am me. One of the nobodies of this world, according to the behavior of many in the medical profession.

Those in the medical profession, physicians, nurses, aids, and others, need to understand they cannot pick or choose who receives better treatment based on their own personal biases. If a physician doesn't click with a person who is seeking medical attention, then that physician should never turn away or terminate the patient/physician relationship without giving a referral of another qualified physician. A physician should never have an attitude or be impossible to work with, or make bad judgment calls such as psychological issues or drug addiction, because of a negative personal opinion.

Medical professionals need to be held accountable for their actions in the medical fields sooner than later. Accountability to adhere by their oath to *First Do No Harm*. If a patient is seeking help and has oddities that may mimic psychological diagnoses or drug addiction symptoms, it is the physicians' responsibility to *First Do No Harm*. The physician IS doing harm by judging and documenting psychological diagnoses and addictions that do not exist. *Accusations Harm*. Physicians need to be held accountable whether they are in the emergency rooms, hospitals, or their personal offices. They decide if you receive treatment or not. As patients, we don't care about the business end of the practice, we care whether we live or die.

I am working to raise funds for research because I know financially, it is impossible to do what needs to be done without the funding. However, the majority of physicians I have seen are not looking for a cure to help someone live; they are spending the 15 minutes that is generally allotted on the schedule, which happens to be the amount of time the insurances use as a guideline to pay the physicians.

How can 15 minutes be a justifiable amount of time for those with extreme difficulties, compared to those who are physically fit and coming in for a checkup? Fifteen minutes is generally enough time to do a checkup on someone who is healthy. What about me? I want to be healthy, but my body refuses to listen to what I tell it to do. I'm not famous, I'm not rich, I haven't won a Pulitzer, but I do things in my life that are as equally important to those I do things for. I wouldn't change who I am for anything in the world. I am happy to be able to finally speak out about so many things that

I have been through to help others. I'm hoping through each book that is written by me or by others, raises the awareness and education needed to help those living with these illnesses. Hopefully everyone will benefit from the knowledge given to live happy healthier lives.

James 1:5-6

If any of you lacks wisdom [to guide him through a decision or circumstance], he is to ask of [our benevolent] God, who gives to everyone generously and without rebuke or blame, and it will be given to him. But he must ask [for wisdom] in faith, without doubting [God's willingness to help], for the one who doubts is like a billowing surge of the sea that is blown about and tossed by the wind.

Chapter 9

Coming to Terms

Regardless of how hard sickness, pain, fatigue or weakness has tried to break my spirit or take my life, I continue to look to God for strength and guidance through this incredibly tough life. Coming to terms with these types of medical issues has been very hard for me. I certainly don't lay around and get down about it. I find a way to keep going while taking rest periods throughout the day. I was once so active. I love life and I love doing things with people and for people. Everywhere I went I always had such a great time. It was easier to smile and laugh then, it didn't hurt as much or take my strength away. Laughter gives you strength in some ways, and in other ways is exhausting when you are not feeling well. I'll take exhaustion from laughter any day over exhaustion from pain and illness.

When I say I don't lay around and let it get me down, I mean I have to lie down or sit down often, but I don't want to let it get me down psychologically, so I keep busy doing positive things I am physically capable of doing.

Of course I get depressed like any other person in the world when something bad happens. I don't stay in that state, but I do get depressed about it at times. I get anxious at times when there is too much on my plate and there is generally never anyone to help me to get through it. It is quite a lot to schedule all of these appointments, see all of these doctors, have all of these health problems, and handle it alone.

People who are sick with any of these Silent Illnesses need everyone's support. Just because you cannot see what is happening, does not mean that person is not telling the truth about the pain, weakness, sickness, and suffering that occurs with any of these illnesses.

Gastroparesis all by itself is painful. Ehlers-Danlos all by itself is painful. Dysautonomia affects the body through our autonomic nervous system. The autonomic nervous system is the system in our body that controls our "fight or flight" responses. For example, when something scares us, our heart rate increases and breathing becomes quick and shallow, in addition to other responses we are not aware of that occur at the same time. When the stimulus that created the fear is gone, our heart slows and our breathing goes back to a normal pace. That is how our bodies should work. With Dysautonomia, the body is unable to follow those normal patterns, creating chronic tachycardia, fainting, insomnia, and so on. Add hormonal imbalances to the mix, and it can feel like the perfect storm. In "Is There a Doctor in the Country? Volume 2," we will go into more detail about the other types of Silent Illnesses, some of which are mentioned above. It is important that everyone knows what is going on in our country with regard to our health, since this is affecting millions.

Our healthcare system is not a system to depend on or trust. Perhaps generations ago you could trust your family doctor to do his best, but not today. Today, money rules this profession, and if you take up too much time, many doctors do not want to accept you into their practice. Too many doctors' offices seem to want the visits to stay short so they can bring in a certain number of patients a day. Too many patients have lost their lives due to ignorance or arrogance. Either one is unacceptable. As patients, we do expect to pay for medical services and have those services be properly rendered. The medical profession is a service industry no different than any other service industry. With one tremendous exception, our lives are being serviced. The lack of medical care, or concern for the patient, can interfere with our ability to live life. When there are so many people living with Gastroparesis, and so few in the medical community who understand anything about the reality of Gastroparesis, many lives become lost under the lack of education and knowledge.

An example of a medical company supplying top quality services to their patients, is the infusion company I use for my IV nutrition and other IV needs at home, Coram Specialty Infusion Services. I have had the same nurse for several years through Coram, as well as the same dietician. I had the same pharmacist until not too long ago. The pharmacist who replaced the one I came to trust is equally as pleasant and helpful to work with. The services provided by this company are top notch. I am treated like I matter, like I am important. The way it should be for everyone, not a selected number. A service is rendered and the person receiving the service pays. In most service professions, we have the right to refuse to pay for bad or unacceptable service. If we have the right as consumers to refuse to pay for inadequate services from other service professions, why are the insurance companies paying for visits to doctors who are not giving us the care required for the health issues we are seeking support for? Or why is it that we get stuck with bills from medical professionals who have not done their job, created another medical bill to add to the collection of growing deductibles, just to pass you off to another doctor who creates another medical bill. It is extremely expensive to be sick. Healthcare costs more in the USA than any other country in the world. You could lose everything if you get sick.

In 2010, 42% of the bankruptcies in the country were due to medical expenses. Of those, 78% had health insurance. There is not enough support for those who are sick with health issues that render them disabled. I have been fighting for my disability for a couple of years because of the lack of knowledge of these illnesses. These illnesses need to be included on a federal level, not to be disputed. The severity of these illnesses have often led to total dependency upon other people, or even death.

Many people judge us when they see us trying to still look good, no matter how we feel. We all have the right to look good if we want to. We shouldn't have to be worried that someone won't believe us just because we don't look sick. On the opposite side, if you go in looking as sick as you feel, you are called a drug seeker because of how horrible you look. There is no winning with so many in the medical profession.

While I know I have all of these medical issues that have no cures, I believe that together, with hard work and perseverance, we can find a cure. Coming to terms with these health problems has been a huge battle for me. I have been researching to find a cure for Gastroparesis since the day I found out what I had. I don't want to die from this. I want to live, play with my granddaughter, go to the movies with my daughter, smell the flowers in the spring and see the beautiful colors in the fall. I want to swim in the Floridian beaches and take a couple of cruises, one of them being the Disney Cruise with my family. I would like to make sure each month, there is an activity of some type to raise money for the research and support of those who are living with these issues. I am a fighter. I always have been. I don't go down very easy, and I thank God for the strength to keep going. I thank God for making me strong, persistent, and compassionate.

Coming to terms for me has taken a number of years. For so many years, I was told all of this was in my head. Being accused of being sick in my head, rather than sick in my body, has been years of outlandish hell. There was validation in one respect with several diagnoses, and an unbelievable feeling of anger toward all of the doctors, over all of these years for not listening to a word I was saying.

As a little girl, I had growing pains so bad, I would be in tears constantly. Growing pains is another word for "I don't know." Not everyone in the world experiences "growing pains." If they were real, everyone would be walking around with them while growing, and that just isn't so. I had so many problems with my health from the time I was young. I wish someone would have taken notice. I know that I don't want to be sick, and I fight hard to stay on my feet and put on a smile. Even though I put a smile on, I know that my body is not doing so well, and many other people who are sick with Silent Illnesses are the same way.

We don't want to be sick so we smile and try to laugh it off in front of people. Behind closed doors, where no one sees the true pain, nausea, and weakness, is where the truth shows itself. Whether I am sick or not, I want to look good. I don't want to look bad, so I make as much effort as possible to put on a smiley face or laugh off what is happening. For me as well, behind closed doors is a different story. That is where very few people are allowed to go. I personally don't want people to see me fighting the pain, nausea, and weakness that I fight. The fatigue that takes my entire body and tries to bring me to my knees along with the rest of the symptoms becomes overwhelming. The only one I can turn to for help is God. There is no one else who can help me get through what I am living with.

There are too many people in this world sick with these types of illnesses, and we have lost too many friends, as well. I haven't come to terms with all of the illnesses that I face every day of my life. I know what I have been diagnosed with, it is just that I don't agree this cannot be changed. I know there are no cures to date, and very few people looking for cures. Very few medical professionals even have an inkling of what any of us are going through, fighting so hard to live. A cure has to be found. Even through natural healthy ways, there has to be something to help. I am going to continue to look for answers to questions and create more questions to answer. I want to know as much as possible about this group of Silent Illnesses so that I have a clearer understanding of how each affects the body. I want to find how to get better now. I don't want anyone to tell me I have to wait years down the road before enough people realize what is happening to work toward finding a cure. I will not accept that either.

What I do expect is that we all have strengths and should stand up together as a united front and fight the injustices related with our healthcare system. United brings a stronger wave of force to create change. One person can bang against a door as long as he wants for help, and his fists are not going to break down that door. But bring a thousand together and two thousand fists, the entire structure will come down where no one can hide from the truth. We need to work together to make sure we receive the support and attention we deserve.

Coming to terms has meant that I take a good look at myself. My life. What I have done, both good and bad. What I should have done differently, and what I had no control over. We all make choices. Right or wrong, they are our choices, and in the end, we all have to live with the choices we make. We have to also learn to forgive ourselves for mistakes we make and learn from them. We cannot go back and change the past. We can only move forward, learning from the past, and making sure to right our wrongs as well as love others as we would ourselves want to be loved. It is important that in this life, we learn to see beyond ourselves. I have had a tough life in many respects. However, if I did not live that life, I would not be able to help others, nor would I be the person I am today.

We are human, and sometimes we hold grudges. Being able to let go of a grudge is imperative in our own growth as individuals. It is possible someone can hurt us so deep, that it may be impossible to form a relationship with that person again. I know all too well that kind of hurt. I also know how important it is to let go of the past. Deep hurt isn't generally forgotten, but it can be forgiven. Even though a hurt can be forgiven, that does not mean a relationship will be mended or continued. People will do what they do. Right or wrong, they will hurt you, let you down, and betray your trust. If we give people too much trust, without being realistic to human flaws, we set ourselves up to be let down.

The important thing is to have that special group of family and friends you know you can trust your dearest secrets with in your life. If your friends and family are the type you cannot trust, make new ones. After all, we only have one life to be happy. We only have one chance to believe in ourselves and love others. We only have one life to be a true friend, and accept a true friend.

Many continue along with their lives, keeping their sunglasses on so they don't have to look at one another. To avoid eye contact means to avoid conversation and life. You never know what smile or kind words you choose that can turn someone else's day around. We live in a world where we all bounce off of one another. In my neighborhood, not many of us make it a point to come out and talk to one another. In my old neighborhood, everyone waved and said, "Hi" and stopped by for an occasional visit. I know for myself, living in that type of neighborhood brought a smile to my heart and my lips.

Again, as I sit here, I wonder if I will ever come to terms with these illnesses. Perhaps not accepting this is coming to terms. I don't know. When you live with something that has tried to take your life on more than one occasion, and you keep pushing forward with *hope*, no matter what things actually look like, every day is a gift. A gift that you want to share with those who are most important to you. So many people walk away from their loved ones when they get sick. Perhaps they cannot handle the idea of death themselves so the thought of watching someone get worse is too much to deal with. I guess that's what people tell themselves. I don't understand where love fits in with that way of thinking.

I'm the type of person who could never give up on someone I love. I could never turn my back on someone I care about. I don't have that capability. If there comes a choice between my welfare, and a family member or friend who may jeopardize my well-being, I will choose myself first. That is not turning my back on someone. That is taking care of myself. Something that took me quite a while to learn.

If someone you love is doing something that can be detrimental to you, no matter what the health scenario, that person unfortunately may not love you, or may not know how to love. Loving and trusting oneself is the best protection we can give ourselves. Trusting ourselves to look for truth in everything, as opposed to believing everything that is said, will always serve us better. Words are cheap where actions speak the truth. I have been through my share of situations where I was not taking care of myself. I was always taking care of everyone else. I've learned I cannot do that anymore. I look back and wish I would have learned this a lot sooner. I should have always put myself first. Not in a selfish way, by being nasty, arrogant, and turning my back on others, but in a loving way. A loving way that keeps peace in our hearts, a spring in our step, and a smile on our face.

Many times we blame others for feelings we have that are ours to deal with, and not for someone else. Our own mindset, our mood, more often than not, is the reason for the outcome of many situations. Whether you are feeling positive or negative, you will reflect onto others the same. Many times people are uncomfortable to be around people who are dealing with medical issues, which in turn may create a negative environment for the person dealing with the health problem. It is so important, especially for close family and friends, to become more accepting of those who have chronic health issues. Become more understanding and compassionate. Generally, the person who is sick doesn't want to be sick. I know for my own self, if I had more supportive, positive people in my life, the degree of difficulty along the way would have decreased. Many who are facing life threatening health issues sometimes feel like they are not as valuable to their family any longer. Coming to terms with health issues, includes family and friends being understanding, compassionate, as well as interested enough to educate themselves on whatever the health issue happens to be. Having family and friends try to understand, as well as be supportive and compassionate, shows someone who is sick they are still important.

###

Psalm 57:1-3

Be merciful to me, O God, be merciful to me! For my soul trusts in You; And in the shadow of Your wings I will make my refuge, until these calamities have passed by. I will cry out to God Most High, to God who performs all things for me. He shall send from heaven and save me…

Chapter 10

Thank You God

From as far back as I can remember, there was never a time when I did not know God was there for me. During these past couple of years, more than ever, I've thought about that quite a bit. It is amazing at times, and so incredible, that there really isn't a time that I have ever doubted God's existence. I may have questioned the order of things at times, but never did I ever doubt God.

My grandparents were two of the most incredible people in my life. They taught me so much about God, Jesus Christ, and the Holy Spirit. Knowing that God is always there with me is comforting. When I call Him, I know He is listening and hears my prayers. I know He knows my tears and hears my laughter. When I stop and look at so much beauty and perfection God has created, I am always amazed and in awe. When it comes to having a relationship with God, and I am not talking about religion, I know with certainty that I am loved and cared for. I can trust in Him no matter what circumstances may seem like. I didn't always know I could trust in Him, and even when I did know, I didn't understand why I faced so many overwhelming obstacles. I see now how each situation made me who I am today. I am stronger to deal with what I am dealing with. Without the strength God created in me, with each trial I have faced, I would not be able to do a fraction of what I am able to do now or then.

As human beings, we ask God for a lot. We ask Him for good health, an honest, caring, loving and devoted spouse, money, a beautiful home, a safe vehicle, help out of a jam, and a million other things. So many people I have spoken with throughout the years, don't want to wait on what God wants. People want what they want, and they want it now, regardless of consequences. If things go wrong, they blame God. If all of their requests aren't granted right away or granted at all, they say God doesn't hear their prayers, or even worse, God doesn't exist. Praying and asking God for something isn't like a magic show. It takes faith, courage, strength, and perseverance to get up every day and trust God, even in the worst situations. Trust Him when you don't see a change, and still continue to trust God every day, until one day you wake up and realize small changes were happening all along. We may not get everything we ask for, but in the end, when we follow where God leads us, we get what we honestly and truly need.

I can look at my own life and see how all of the things I've lived through, from the time I was a small child, have come together for my good, and the good of others. It sure didn't feel good going through so much of what I have, but now I can see how so many challenges and difficulties prepared me to fight this fight and help others along the way. I know every day is a blessing, and there are many reasons I should not be alive. I only have God to thank for that. The only way I can get up every day is by God's grace and mercy. My body doesn't work very well, which is not a pessimistic comment, but a realistic one. Most days I'm housebound or bedbound. Many days I have spent in the hospital. I have fewer good days physically than difficult days, but I am grateful for every moment. I feel like God wants me to tell people what He has done for me. I have fought so many life threatening complications, and been through so much in my life because of my health, I want people to know how much He has done for me. God has shown me, through so many incredible miracles, that He has been right there with me the entire way.

I didn't feel like it was my responsibility to tell people about God. For a long time, I didn't think God loved me enough. I didn't think I was special. When I was in middle school, my very good friend went to church with me one Sunday. We were in the 8th grade and getting ready to move up to high school. It was the first year 9th grade students were schooled with the high school students. The church I went to when I was younger, was a church that believed in the gift of tongues. A language spoken between the Holy Spirit and our spirit. I believe in the gift of tongues, but I know I have seen a number of people who were not honest about actually being blessed with the gift. I watched people put on a show when I was little, and I could tell the difference. God has blessed me with beautiful gifts, I am so honored to have. While that may not have been one of my gifts at the time my friend came with me to church, I was respectful of those who did have that gift and used it during the wonderful singing time of praise. I do love singing songs of praise. I love it today in my own church, which is a community church that reaches out to so many.

Anyway, that Sunday night when I went to bed, I had no idea what was waiting around the corner. I called my friend the next day, and her mother told me I was never allowed to talk to her or play with her again. I was devastated. I could not believe that my good friend, who I had so many fun times with, was being ripped out of my life. The tears I cried. The pain I went through. I could not believe that someone could be so cruel. During our high school education, when you move up with your friends, I ended up being one of the kids who didn't have many friends in school to move up with. The one good friend I thought I had, I wasn't even allowed to speak to anymore, and she never spoke a word to me. During high school, she passed me by as if she never knew who I was. That hurt too. I guess I could have never done something like that to someone, and I could not believe that God had let someone do that to me. I came to realize over the years that you don't necessarily end up where you think you are going in this life. God's plans always supersede our own.

I believe it is a privileged to be here, every second of every day. Along the road in my life, there have been so many obstacles. Had I not survived all that I did, had I not screamed and yelled at God at times, had I not called to Him wondering if He was really there, I know I would not have made it this far. I would not be here today writing this book if God wasn't real. I would not have done a lot of things I was able to do if it wasn't for the strength He gave me. I am proud to know God loves me this much; that He carried me through so that I could give back to others. Life is hard, but without God and love, life can be so much worse. Even when I was alone and isolated, and on my worst days of being sick, God was always there.

I believe it is important to thank God for everything, the good and the bad. We learn a lesson every time we go through some type of a challenge or life altering experience. Too many get caught up in the game of money, and forget the world around them. It is frustrating to watch how wrapped up people are in money and popularity, while so many people living with health issues like I do. We cannot jump into the rat race of working, fighting to get to the top first. We do what we can from our computers. Most of the time our only connection to the outside world is through our computers. I have been able to research Gastroparesis and related illnesses over the past couple years, through the Internet, sharing the information with others who have these illnesses. I will continue to post research on GastroparesisAndME.com, and GPNMEGlobal.org, as well as my main Facebook page @Tanya.L.Taylor.

I thank God for all of the incredible people He has put in my life. All of the people I have learned to call friend. All of those who are there for me, and I am able to be there for them as well. I don't believe we are to be alone in this world. I believe we are all a piece of one giant puzzle. There is one thing I have learned and will never forget: Life is like a rose garden, so many beautiful flowers and life to behold, and so many thorns to get through. It is important to always see the beauty in the midst of the thorns, to always "Stop and Smell the Roses." Unless we can appreciate the beauty through all of the hard times, we get drawn into the difficulties and lose sight of the bigger picture. Don't be afraid to love with all of your heart. Everyone needs someone. That is just how we are made. Even the meanest of people usually have someone they turn to, regardless of the validity of that relationship.

I thank God for my incredible daughter, Sam. She has and always will be the beat of my heart. As a parent, I've made my share of mistakes, and have hurt my daughter without realizing how much I had. Living as sick as I have, has also been a great fear on Sam's heart that a child should not have to bear. However, it has been through this illness that I have come to see so clearly how important it is to put God first in all decisions. This life is only temporary. I thank God every day for my incredible granddaughter, Carissa. She is a joy, a wonderful and amazing little girl. Throughout Carissa's life, she too has seen me carted off to the hospital by ambulance on multiple occasions from fever spikes, blood infections, internal bleeding, and other complications since she was born. While we can dwell on the multiple negative circumstances and sometimes life threatening health problems, we choose to thank God for getting through to be here another day. While this life is so very painful and debilitating, my family still depends on me. I want to be there for them as much as I can before it is my time to go home. I believe God carries me through this rocky storm so that I may be a blessing to my family, and others. My girls are the blood in my veins, and have taken me through some incredible journeys of the heart. Without those incredible experiences, as wonderful as some were and as difficult as others were, I would never have learned as much about life and love as I have. I learned so much about myself. Sam is the one who showed me how important it is to let things go so you can be free to love those in your life.

Life is too short. We are only here for a blink of an eye, and then we are gone. Believing in something you cannot see is only difficult when you don't have *faith*. I thank God every day for having *faith* to continue on this journey, despite the physical hardships and challenges that I have to face. I thank God for the family and friends I have in my life. God Bless Everyone. We need it in this world we live in today.

###

Isaiah 40:28-31

Hast thou not known? Hast thou not heard, that the everlasting God, the Lord, the Creator of the ends of the earth, never grows faint, never grows weary? There is no searching of His understanding. He giveth power to the faint, and to them that have no power, He gives them strength. Even the youths shall fain and grow weary, and young men will fall; but those that wait upon the Lord shall renew their strength; they shall mount up with wings as eagles, they shall run and not be weary, and they shall walk and not faint.

Chapter 11

Understanding Gastroparesis

Gastroparesis technically means paralysis of the gastric system. Gastric, according to definition from the Merriam-Webster Dictionary means, "of or relating to the stomach." Medline Plus, a service of the U.S. National Library of Medicine, NIH, also uses Merriam-Webster Dictionary, Medical, for that and other definitions. MediLexicon defines Gastric as "relating to stomach." Gastroparesis is a Digestive Tract Paralysis Disorder. The National Digestive Disease Information Clearinghouse's (NDDIC) definition of *Gastroparesis, also called delayed gastric emptying, is a disorder that slows or stops the movement of food from the stomach to the small intestine. Normally, the muscles of the stomach, which are controlled by the vagus nerve, contract to break up food and move it through the gastrointestinal (GI) tract. The GI tract is a series of hollow organs joined in a long, twisting tube from the mouth to the anus. The movement of muscles in the GI tract, along with the release of hormones and enzymes, allows for the digestion of food. Gastroparesis can occur when the vagus nerve is damaged by illness or injury and the stomach muscles stop working normally. Food then moves slowly from the stomach to the small intestine or stops moving altogether.* PubMed Health, which is related to the National Institute of Health (NIH), provides this definition of Gastroparesis, *"Gastroparesis is a condition that reduces the ability of the stomach to empty its contents. It does not involve a blockage (obstruction)."* Mayo Clinic's definition, *"Gastroparesis is a condition in which the muscles in your stomach don't function normally."* The Ohio State University gives this definition, *"Gastroparesis is a stomach disorder in which the stomach takes too long in emptying its contents. If food remains in the stomach for too long, it can cause problems such as bacterial overgrowth from the fermentation of the food. The food can also harden into solid masses, called bezoars, that may cause nausea, vomiting, and, sometimes, obstruction in the stomach. This can be dangerous if they block the passage of food into the small intestine."* WebMD's definition is, *"Gastroparesis is a condition in which your stomach cannot empty itself of food in a normal fashion. It is caused by damage to the vagus nerve, which regulates the digestive system. A damaged vagus nerve prevents the muscles in the stomach and intestine from functioning, preventing food from moving through the digestive system properly. Often, the cause of gastroparesis is unknown."*

Each one of the five definitions contain the word "stomach." Each one of the definitions refers to Gastroparesis as being a problem with the stomach muscles being able to move and empty the stomach, or a problem with the stomach emptying. In three definitions, the vagus nerve, or nerve X, is mentioned as a probable reason for the problem with muscle function. In one definition, the words "digestive system" are used, and in one definition, "gastrointestinal (GI) tract" is used. These definitions come from some of the top medical locations in our country. It is important to see the vagueness or clarity words can bring. By suggesting the stomach muscles are the main culprit for Gastroparesis, to someone who knows little or nothing about this silent illness, it does not bring to light that the rest of the digestive system may be compromised and can actually be a part of the problem with the stomach not emptying properly. Some of the other parts of the digestive system below the stomach include the pyloric sphincter, duodenum, jejunum, ileum, ascending colon, transverse colon, descending colon, cecum, rectum, anus, as well as the pancreas, liver and gall bladder that can be contributing to the sluggish movement to paralyzed state of the stomach. Should the colon not be functioning from Colonic Inertia, it can reduce the ability for the stomach to empty into the small intestine, if the colon is not functioning and cannot empty what is backing up in the digestive system. A colon with Colonic Inertia acts as a plug in the digestive system. There are some who believe that the stomach emptying cannot be affected by Colonic Inertia. I know that it is 100% the truth because I lived it, had my colon removed after the perforation, and survived it. My stomach starting emptying right after that surgery, so there is no doubt. The rest of the system slowed up as time continued, but the plug created by the colon was gone after the surgery to remove it.

Not in any of the definitions for Gastroparesis, do I see where any of the other parts of the digestive system are mentioned as being culprits for the decreased motility or lack of motility, in the gastric (stomach) area. When my colon was removed, I could eat again for a little while. So the way I see things with my own body, is that my digestive system is slowly stopping from the colon up through the rest of my digestive tract. My small intestine now feels identical to how my colon did as it was slowly ceasing to function, resulting in a perforation. I worry at times that my small intestine may rupture or perforate because of the pain and constant problem in the lower right quadrant of my abdomen, the upper center and the left side mid abdomen.

Over the past couple of years, through asking questions to people who have Gastroparesis, it seems like the digestive system is either negatively affected from the stomach down, or from the colon up. By this I mean that the constipation from the colon not functioning, blocks the system from functioning properly. It slows down the small intestine and stomach from functioning properly, not allowing the contents of the food to move through. Or, the stomach's inability to push the foods through the pyloric valve into the duodenum, the beginning part of the small intestine, and then into the jejunum, the next part of the small intestine. In that situation, a gastric pacer may decrease nausea, allowing someone to continue to take food in by mouth. In other circumstances, a Jtube may be inserted to the small intestine or GJtube may be inserted into the stomach and then into the small intestine, to bypass the stomach.

Colonic Inertia is a condition that I suffered with for years. This led to the removal of my colon, approximately three feet in length. The colon is part of the digestive system. After my colon was removed, my stomach was moving and I was able to eat food again. The definition for Colonic Inertia, by the Digestive Disease Center says *"Some people suffer from severe abdominal pain because their colon holds on to feces too long. They generally do not complain of difficulty emptying their rectum. Instead, they feel as if their intestinal contents never get to their rectum. If there is nothing else found to be the cause of their symptoms, these people may suffer from colonic inertia ... a colon that pumps too slowly."* It is difficult to find an exact definition, but there are more lengthy explanations of what is defined by the Digestive Disease Center. I know after living with Colonic Inertia, you have no idea what constipation pain feels like, until you have been constipated for 14 days.

A nurse told my daughter, during an emergency room visit, that she knows how painful it is to be constipated. My daughter was well beyond constipated. She had not gone in 12 days. When she was finally able to go to the bathroom, the poisonous smell that filled the air of the entire house was so bad, we had to open all of the windows to breathe. The contrast that the hospital gave, which is a liquid that a patient drinks to light up the inside during the CT, is what eventually helped her bowels release. The CT showed she was compacted, but then she was sent home with a diagnosis of constipation. An intestine this compacted can surely perforate or rupture. Eventually, if something doesn't give, the body won't be able to stay in that compacted state forever. This type of pain feels like your intestines are going to rupture, because that is exactly what could happen. They are being stretched too far, with old food that is not moving and turning to poison in our bodies. This is one of the reasons constipation can create such overwhelming gas smells. It becomes toxic after sitting for days in the intestinal tract.

Colonic Inertia can cause perforations of the colon. I have not personally spoken with someone who has had a colonic rupture, but I have read about the possibility of this happening. I had a colonic perforation which also dumps poison into your system in the same way a rupture does. Either way, should this happen, this type of poison in our systems will lead to death if not treated

215

right away. I know about this first hand. I have read how rare a perforation or rupture is, but is it that rare with these illnesses? I don't know. I think doing some research would be necessary to find an answer that would satisfy me. So many studies and reports use data that is supposed to be a representative of the population as a whole. I don't see how that is possible when there are so many people who do not seek medical treatment for various reasons. There are too many parts of the population that are not considered in several studies I had read, not only with Colonic Inertia, but with Gastroparesis as well. I personally think it is important to do a more in depth research study that counts the heads of all of those in each state. Those who are diagnosed with Gastroparesis, those who are in the process of being diagnosed, and those who are symptomatic and have no idea what is happening. Without that data, it is impossible to know how many people are really sick with these medical issues.

I would like to put together a study, collect the data needed to find out how many people actually have these health issues, but the amount of man power it would take to collect that information costs quite a bit more than I personally have to spend. Writing for funding to do this type of a program would be the only way to offset the costs. It would provide part time work to a few people in each one of the states, until all of the data is collected. The information, I believe would prove to be invaluable, and the protection of so many people who are suffering with the consequences of these Silent Illnesses.

In our country, there is always talk about "family" and "quality of life." Whether in the news or a political campaign, we hear how important it is for each person to have equal opportunity to have a good "quality of life" and be part of your "family." However, it takes two incomes to meet the ever growing costs of the basic needs of a family; and the ability to participate in your own "family" becomes extremely difficult, if not impossible depending upon the work schedule. When you add in unexpected illnesses or medical complications, your "quality of life" diminishes and the family suffers. If there isn't a way to make up the extra income needed to offset the extra costs, either the family loses everything they had prior to the onset of the health issues, or someone has to work two full time jobs and is never able to participate in their own family life. If family is as important as the government says it is, and media says it is, then why are so many families trying to figure out how to pay their rents or mortgages, go to the grocery store to eat, and pay for medical needs when someone in the family gets too sick? Many illnesses diminish a person's "quality of life" and while every person has the right to have their basic needs met, many go without and are treated subhuman in so many ways. This should not be happening. Too many people are judged by their appearance, and many people with this group of silent illnesses do not look sick.

My "quality of life" during my twenties and thirties along with my daughter's, led me to make rash decisions I may not have made otherwise. I created my own business to live, because I was too sick to work for someone else. My body does not tolerate sitting behind a desk, and working at a computer for any length of time. While writing this book, I have to stop, move around, do something else and then come back to it. I have to lie down or sit in different positions to be able to type and research from the laptop. My neck and back cannot take the constant stressful position of a desk. My shoulders have gotten to a point they cannot take much pressure so I cannot lean on them much, and have to watch my positioning. I have Ehlers-Danlos, a connective tissue disorder, to thank for that. There is not enough known about Ehlers-Danlos either. They do know there are different types and that the collagen breaks down.

Collagen makes the skin tight, the blood vessels strong, and the connective tissue near the joints strong enough to hold the bones in place. With the breakdown of our collagen, our joints are compromised, vessels weakened, skin loosened and stretchy, and our muscles have to do more work than they would if everything was alright. Ehlers-Danlos also causes problems with the joints, skin, skeletal system, digestive system, memory, and more.

Along this journey, finding out there are so many different Silent Illnesses has been mind blowing. My mind cannot grasp the fact that there are this many people sick, with little known or discussed. There are many people who are extremely symptomatic, however, there are not enough people in the medical field educated, or required to learn about this group of Silent Illnesses, that includes Gastroparesis, so that so many people are not overlooked and misdiagnosed.

"Is There a Doctor in the Country? Volume 2" will have more detailed information about Ehlers-Danlos, Dysautonomia, Chiari Malformation, and Mast Cell Activation Disorders. Silent Illnesses result in too many people unable to work to provide for their families. They also cause missed time from work or school, the inability to spend quality time with your family, costly medical bills, or no medical care due to the inability to afford it. Join me, in Volume 2, and a couple of other people, who will share their journey while surviving and living with these Silent Illnesses.

Isaiah 58:11

And the Lord will guide you continually and satisfy your desire in scorched places and make your bones strong; and you shall be like a watered garden, like a spring of water, whose waters do not fail.

Chapter 12

What You Can Do

There are many things each one of us can do when it comes to support. Be understanding, and show patience to the person living with this devastating illness. Spread awareness in any common or unique way possible. Help to raise funds for research and support of those who are reaching out to organizations for help. Show kindness to those who are living with these illnesses, and any other type of illness for that fact.

Many people who are sick with chronic health issues, do not look sick. Many do not live in a wheelchair, hospital bed, or other type of assisted equipment. Many people get up every day, go to work, no matter how they are feeling, and make the best of it while trying to find a cure. Many people are unable to function or get out of the house without assistance, and often end up alone.

The people who need assistance to live with Gastroparesis and related illnesses do not generally look sick, but need as much help as someone fighting a devastating cancer.

There are times I can get my hair together, a little bit of make-up on, an outfit appropriate for an event, and look radiant. To do that, I have to get ready in increments of time, doing only a small bit at a time to get myself ready, resting in between, while getting some help from Mike. However, I still need the assistance of someone to help me get out of the house and to the event, as well as get through the event, even if it is only for an hour, and then get me home. Having assistance would allow me to function, and actually go somewhere outside of my own home. It is good to have the support of someone who tries to be understanding. The amount of support we need, when we are feeling our worst, is a lot of work. If I am out, I may suddenly become sick and need help getting to the bathroom to throw up, or have a sweltering hot flash that causes me to have tachycardia, dizziness, shortness of breath, as well as the possibility of passing out. Life can become very interesting at times. A shoulder to lean on may be needed more than anything else.

To have someone try to be a friend when living with something that makes you this sick, is a rarity. People seem to stay more to themselves than want to reach out. Community members, on a larger scale, are encouraged to become more active through associations, community centers, schools, churches, and so on. So why, on a smaller scale, in our own neighborhoods, is there not more encouragement of interactions and support? Why do we participate in larger scale community activities, but in our own neighborhoods, we often fail to be friendly neighbors? Our society today seems to dictate that we do for ourselves, get as much as we can for ourselves, and then we will be happy. Just look on television at the commercials. I think that speaks for itself.

We all have our own lives, and we are all busy, but do we have to be so busy that we cannot check on our neighbors we know are sick, or check on our neighbors who have just had a baby, or a death in the family, and so on? So many people put blinders on when they pull into their own neighborhood? I'm guilty of doing it myself. I don't want to be that way, however, on most days, I am not feeling well and completely drained of energy. On so many days my body does what it wants to do, making it nearly impossible to get out and associate with anyone. There are times I can put on the "I'm Ok" face, while pushing through just to be able to say Hi, but for the most part, it takes everything out of me just to walk out of my front door.

Often times, family members are not understanding of a family member who is sick with a chronic illness. Especially one you cannot see. We need our families to realize that not everyone has the energy to get their body moving, driving, working, exercising, or participating in any other normal daily life activity. We often do not look as bad as we feel, so I think many family members do not understand that we feel as awful as we do. When people in our families get sick, more often than not, they become more understanding of our struggles, as well as sorry we have to go through so much.

Mike twisted his ankle one time. I didn't want him to be hurt, but I was so upset with him. He was hobbling, and huffing, and grunting for a couple of days, while I have no choice but to live in a daily torture chamber without any escape. I was able to get him a few things he needed the first day, and a little help on the second day, but I couldn't help much more than that. I thought about all of the help I needed while I was home alone every day, six days a week, all year long. I needed so much care most of the time that I ended up in bed waiting for help, while Mike worked six days a week, every week. Living with

Gastroparesis, Ehlers-Danlos, Dysautonomia, and Mast Cell Disorder, makes it incredibly difficult to get through a day alone. Most of the time, Mike doesn't think about the energy and effort it takes for me just to get up in the morning and brush my teeth, let alone everything it will take out of me to get through an entire day. I have needed so much more support than I have had. I truly believe that if I would have had more support, I would have been able to focus more on taking care of myself, which would have given me more energy to spend quality time with my family doing something fun. The only way to make arrangements that will benefit everyone in the family is to work together. It may be upsetting and frustrating to figure out how to best make things work for everyone, but it is necessary in order to get through this life of chronic illness.

When Mike hurt his ankle, I asked him how he would be able to get through a day, if something happened increasing his ankle pain so high, that it soared throughout his entire body making it impossible to move without assistance. Then I asked him how he would feel if he told me exactly the help he needed, but I told him I didn't want to hear about it and walked away. I asked him how he would feel if I completely ignored his cries of pain, instead of doing something to help him get comfortable. I lived that way for years. No one believed I was sick, even after the colon perforated and was removed. No one cared that I needed to find doctors who knew what was happening to me, so that I could live my life the best I could as well. By walking away and not caring, too many years were wasted and too many people got hurt. I know we are not the first married couple to face chronic illness, and we definitely will not be the last. But I do know firsthand the importance of your spouse giving you the respect of living a life with health problems so debilitating, so physically devastating, you are unable to do the smallest of tasks. You no longer have a life of choices. You are trapped in a body that you need to make adjustments with everything you do. Having someone love you and respect you regardless of what is happening, is what real love is made of.

If you are not sick, but have hurt yourself so bad that you will never forget that pain, imagine that pain never stopping. Imagine having to live with that every day, but add bouts of increasing pain, along with weakness, nausea, and vomiting. On top of that, imagine there is no cure, and it will only get worse. Most people don't understand what all of the different types of cancer do, but when you say the word cancer, they stop. This is no different. Many people have lost their lives. Many people are still fighting for their lives with no cure in sight. I am one of them. So is my daughter and granddaughter. Unless our families and friends understand us, how will the rest of the world?

In this life, many of us have a gradual increase of problems, while some of us have a tremendous increase of problems at once. Gastroparesis and related illnesses are different for everyone, as well as so many similarities. When we have an increase in problems, it feels like we take another step down. We have no choice but to adjust and learn to live with whatever extra is added to our plate. Pain makes anyone irritable, but right now, those in my life doesn't seem to understand or appreciate that. I try to live happy, but it's hard when everyone wants you to be more than you are. More than what you have become. No one wants to lose their ability to be independent and have fun. It is so important to have the understanding and compassion from family and friends to make this life a bit easier to live. It gets hard just to sit alone every day and try to meditate the pain away. Nausea and vomiting makes anyone want to stay in and not go out and socialize. Think of it like this, if you have a bad case of food poisoning that would not go away, would you want to go out and have fun with friends and family? Weakness and fatigue makes anyone who wants to live, have no choice but to fight for everything they do. The entire process is exhausting, but much more doable with the support from those around us to help lessen the load of the ups and downs. It would allow so many people to live their lives the best they can, regardless of what stage they are at.

I know for me personally, if I had someone helping me with what I needed to do throughout the day, I know I would actually be able to function to a degree that maybe I could cook sometimes, or do a load of laundry. People living with these illnesses do not want their responsibilities to disappear, but cannot physically keep up as medical issues increase. It is hurtful to have others say mean things to you about not being able to take care of your home or family anymore. It is hard to lose the ability to carry out daily activities when we become sicker. When someone is constantly being critical of what you can and cannot do, it is an unbearable hurt. A hurt that I have seen push people to the point of suicide. I pray I reach families who need to be more understanding of the difficulties we face every day. I pray such a change takes place in families across the Globe, that these devastating health issues can no longer be hidden from the public eye. That families who do not understand what is happening, begin to understand and become that strength and support we need to lean on. That our families help us in leading this march to end the devastating and torturous life we are forced to live, and change it.

People live on the edge of giving up when the pain and suffering becomes too great. This illness may not be understood yet, but that does not mean it is not as devastating and debilitating as we are letting everyone know it is. I pray the silence that hovers over those with Gastroparesis and related illnesses is broken, and answers are found. Like the winds in a hurricane, we need the momentum and support of everyone to help us in our fight for protection from the lack of education and misdiagnosing. It is imperative that the education of these particular Silent Illnesses becomes a topic as well-known as cancer, Lupus, HIV/AIDS, and so on. We need everyone to stand up and take notice that we are out here fighting as hard as we can to survive, and make some kind of life out of what we have been given. This country is always talking about the importance of family and community. It is well past time that this country walks the talk.

I sometimes imagine a world where people actually smile, even when things are going wrong. Where people care about people, regardless of what their situation is. Judgment about appearances disappear, and replaced with fresh eyes to see that not everyone can do everything someone else can do. We are all different, with different strengths and attributes. What a world that would be. A world where it is ok to be different.

2 Corinthians 5:21

He made Christ who knew no sin to [judicially] be sin on our behalf, so that in Him we would become the righteousness of God [that is, we would be made acceptable to Him by His gracious loving kindness].

Chapter 13

A Special Thank You

There are many people I would like to thank for being there for me throughout many times in my life when I felt so alone. I don't want to forget anyone and I apologize if I do. So with that being said, thank you to all of my GP friends, EDS friends, and Dysautonomia friends. Without your support and understanding, I think I may be bald from pulling out my hair, or worse. After I found out my diagnosis of Gastroparesis in 2011, I started to look for other people who had this illness. I had no idea the number of people I would find, or the support I would find, that has kept me fighting on so many occasions.

I have made many friends through so many support systems that were developed by people who are also sick. When there is nothing available, the only thing left to do is create it. Develop something for people with Gastroparesis and related illnesses to be able to go for support, to be understood. When I first began looking for support, there were only a few places to visit online. Now, there are so many different support groups online, take your pick. It is wonderful. Thank you to each group that has been created to provide support.

To my best friend, Sue, thank you for being there to listen those many days and nights of tears and tough times. Thank you for years of fun and good times while we were growing up. We have known one another since grade school, and throughout those years we have had countless laughs and crazy times. I'm glad it was you who was there.

To my friend Pam, thank you for helping me with healthy products I was unfamiliar with, so that I could add them to my daily routine and find some relief. You were so welcoming when I came over to your home, and became such a caring and supportive friend. I am very fortunate to have met you, and have had so many wonderful times together. I'm looking forward to bringing Carissa up with me to see everyone after I heal from surgery. She misses you, and she misses Charlie too. She's ready to play ball. See you soon. Thank you.

To my mother, thank you for driving me to Philadelphia, PA and to Washington, DC, after picking me up from Howard County, MD first. Her initial leaving point from her house was in a different part of Pennsylvania, about an hour and 20 minutes away from my home. Thank you for coming and helping additional times when you were able to come. A couple of times you came over, there was no way I was able to get out of bed. It would have been a horrible day if you were not there. Thank you.

Thank you Dr. Mehran Habibi, for removing my colon and being concerned for my quality of life after surgery. You did everything you could so that I did not end up with a colostomy bag.

Thank you Dr. Clair Francomano for taking the time to listen to what I had to say. Thank you for thoroughly checking me over and answering questions that I have had for decades, and for diagnosing me. By diagnosing me, not only can I tell other doctors this is not in my head, but you have made it possible for my daughter and granddaughter to receive real help from the medical community and not live through the experiences I have had to. Thank you for referring me to Dr Fraser Henderson. Without you, none of the care I am finally receiving would have been possible.

Thank you Dr. Fraser Henderson for finding the reason for my deteriorating muscles, and taking care of my neck to fix the problem, along with all of the others the surgery will fix. Thank you for referring me to Bethesda Physiocare where I had the great privilege of meeting Dr.

Maria Arini. Thank you for listening to me and not turning me away, as so many have done in the past. Thank you for helping me be able to get my life back.

Thank you Dr. Maria Arini for listening to everything I had to say, as well as asking me more questions to be able to properly treat me. Thank you for the dry needling therapy sessions. You have given me new *hope*. Thank you for laughing with me through some of this to make the situation a little easier. Thank you for taking the time to listen and work on my stomach first. Without you, I would not have started to regain some of my life back. It was at the very end of this book that you began the dry needling. I will be discussing this in the second book in the series. This is truly the start of a new life for me. Thank you.

Thank you to my friend Sue in Florida, and her entire family. Thank you for letting me stay with you when I came to visit alone. Thank you all for making room for me and treating me like one of the family. Thank you Sue for being on the phone, listening to the doctors and helping me speak out during one of the most nerve-racking hospital stays I have had. Thank you, and your family, for being supportive, caring, and kind.

Thank you to my friend, Cathi, for being there for the past 14 years or so. Having you as a friend has meant more than you probably realize. You were there when I felt horrible and had to run my own business. You were there when I was having such difficulty getting through the days from the severe pain and nausea, as well as the exhaustion during the time I was taking care of my grandmom while being a single parent. You were there as a calm quiet comfort. You have helped me, and continue to help me, get through some exceptionally tough times. You have seen me at some of my worst times, but never once did you say you did not want to be around me because it was too much for you to handle. Thank you.

Thank you to Cathi's son, Corey for creating the Gastroparesis and ME logo, which will become the GPnME Global, Inc. logo, when I had too much on my plate to even begin to be creative. I know I wanted something unique and you nailed it! Thank you for helping me in and out when I come over, without a second thought or even a moment of hesitation. You are a special young man.

Thank you to Cathi's son, Ian, for being there to carry things and help me out when my body wouldn't let me have the independence or strength to carry things alone. Thank you for the smiles and lighthearted laughter. You are a special young man as well.

To my daughter, Sam. Thank you for being you. Thank you for the 23 years of life I have had with you, and the nine months I carried you. Thank you for snuggling with me when you were a teenager, and holding my hand. When you were little, you were a Mama's girl and those were the

242

best days of my life. I loved the way you called me *Mama* and smiled at me with your beautiful blue eyes. I loved taking you everywhere with me. We were joined at the hip. Thank you for being my daughter, bringing my beautiful granddaughter into this world, and for throwing that heating pad on me when that fever hit. I love you very much, and I always will. You are my *Baby Girl*.

Thank you to my granddaughter, Carissa for being Grandma's *Big Girl* who I love so so much. Thank you for all of your smiles and laughs, all of the love and snuggles. Thank you for watching movies with me and wanting me to play with you out back on the swing set. I love watching you ride your motor scooter out front, and ride your bike. Reading your Children's Bible to you each night has been so special for Grandma. You know so many stories of the Bible and love to talk about them. Each night Grandma has read to you, you end up falling asleep while I am reading. I love to watch you sleep sweetheart. You are such an angel. Just like your Mommy. *I love you and your mommy more than all the skies and all the trees.*

To my husband, Mike. Thank you. We have been through so much. We had so many good times before I had to have my colon removed. While I know so many years were so hard, I believe God is bigger than anything else we can imagine. I believe He holds our lives in His hands, and no matter what we have been through, He will see us through the rest of the way. Having you come to church with me has been more special to me than you can imagine. I love spending that time with you. I wouldn't want anyone but you to stand by my side. No matter what the past has held for us, I believe our future has more good in store for us than either you or I can comprehend. I know it has been scary. I'm the one fighting, but I cannot imagine watching you go through what I have. I know there have been times I may have not made it through, putting your heart through a shredder. No matter how hard things have been for us through this crazy Gastroparesis life, I'm looking forward to the rest of our lives because I believe God uses all things for our good. You will always have my heart. I love you.

To everyone, may God bless you and keep you safe during all of your trials and storms.

###

John 10:10

The Thief comes only in order to steal and kill and destroy. I came that they may have and enjoy life, and hit it in abundance [to the full, till it overflows].

Information Sources

A.D.A.M. Medial Encyclopedia [Internet].
A.D.A.M., Inc; ©2013. Gastroparesis;

[Last reviewed 2012 Oct 8]; [about 1p]. Available
from:

http://www.ncbi.nlm.nih.gov/pubmedhealth/PMH
0001342/   (2013 Mar)

Keith-Ferris, Jeanne, RN, BScN [Internet]. (Aug
19, 2003). Gastroparesis and Related

Digestive MotilityDiseases, a Medical Crisis.
Retrieved from

http://www.digestivedistress.com/sites/default/file
s/pdf/White_Paper_%20on_GI_moitility_diseases
_GPDA_submis.pdf (2012 Aug)

Hoogerwerf WA, Pasricha PJ, Kalloo AN, Shuster
MM [Internet]. (April 1999). Pain: the overlooked
symptom in gastroparesis. The American Journal

of Gastroenterology. [1999 April, 94(4): 1029-33].
Retrieved from
http://www.ncbi.nlm.nih.gov/pubmed/10201478
(2013 Mar)

National Digestive Diseases Information
Clearinghouse [Internet]. (June 2012). What is

Gastroparesis? NIH Publication No. 12-4348.
[June 2012]. Retrieved from
http://www.digestive.niddk.nih.gov/ddiseases/pub
s/gastroparesis/#1 (2012 Nov)

Mayo Clinic Staff [Internet]. (Jan 4 2012).
Gastroparesis Definition. Retrieved from

http://www.mayoclinic.org/diseases-
conditions/gastroparesis/basics/definition/con-
20023971 (May 2012).

WebMD [Internet]. ©2012. What is
Gastroparesis? [Reviewed by Melinda Ratini, DO,
MS on

August 14, 2012]. Retrieved from
http://www.webmd.com/digestive-disorders/digestive-disorders-gastroparesis (Sept 2012).

Health Insure [Internet]. ©2013. Flexible Spending Accounts Useful For Health Expense Savings. Retrieved from
http://www.healthinsure.org/flexible-spending-accounts-useful-for-health-expense-savings/ (Jan 2014).

Support and Resource Links for Patients

Gastroparesis and ME, LLC

http://www.GastroparesisAndME.com (Fiscally Sponsored while

GP and ME obtains 501c3 Nonprofit Status)

ZeroPoint Global

http://www.ttaylor.zeropointglobal.com

Gastroparesis and ME FB Page

https://www.facebook.com/gpandmeglobal

Inspire internet support group

https://www.inspire.com

MDJunction internet support group

http://www.mdjunction.com

Emily's Stomach FB support group

http://www.facebook.com/emilysstomach

Gastroparesis People Helping Each Other FB support group

https://www.facebook.com/groups/Gastropeop lehelping/

Laughing Through Gastroparesis

https://www.facebook.com/groups/laughingthrugp/

Gastroparesis FB support group

https://www.facebook.com/groups/214716548576248/

The Ehlers-Danlos National Foundation

http://www.ednf.org

Ehlers-Danlos (and all related disorders) support group

https://www.facebook.com/groups/336386379826366/

But You Don't Look Sick FB support group

https://www.facebook.com/groups/Butyoudontlooksick/

The ILC Foundation in Canada

http://www.theilcfoundation.org/

Is There A Doctor In The Country?